PERSEVERANCE AND PASSION:

THE PEOPLE WHO SHAPED HEALTH CARE

IN UKIAH, CALIFORNIA

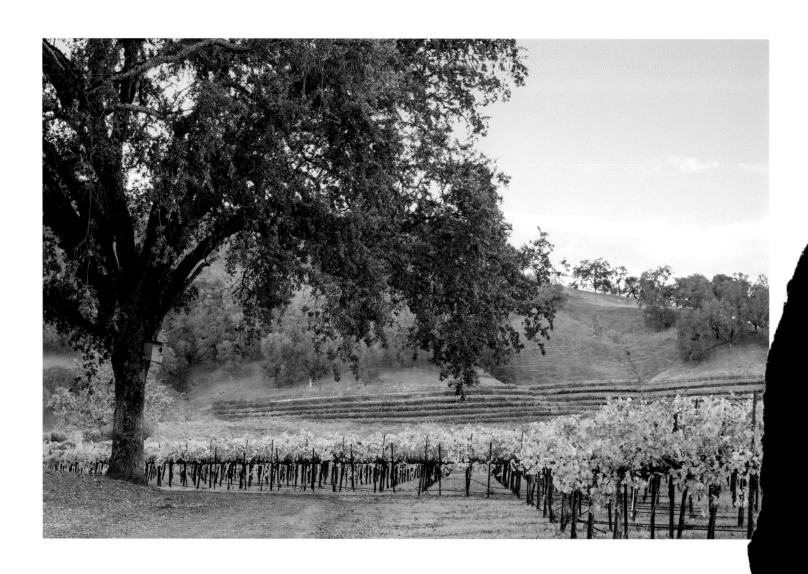

PERSEVERANCE & PASSION

The People Who Shaped Health Care in Ukiah, California

Jendi Coursey

UKIAH VALLEY MEDICAL CENTER

UKIAH, CALIFORNIA

2016

Published by
Ukiah Valley Medical Center
275 Hospital Drive
Ukiah, California 95482

ISBN 13: 978-0 9976386-7-7 (CLOTH EDITION)
ISBN 13: 978-0-9976386-6-0 (SOFT COVER)

First edition

Printed in Canada

Table of Contents

Table of Contents, continued...

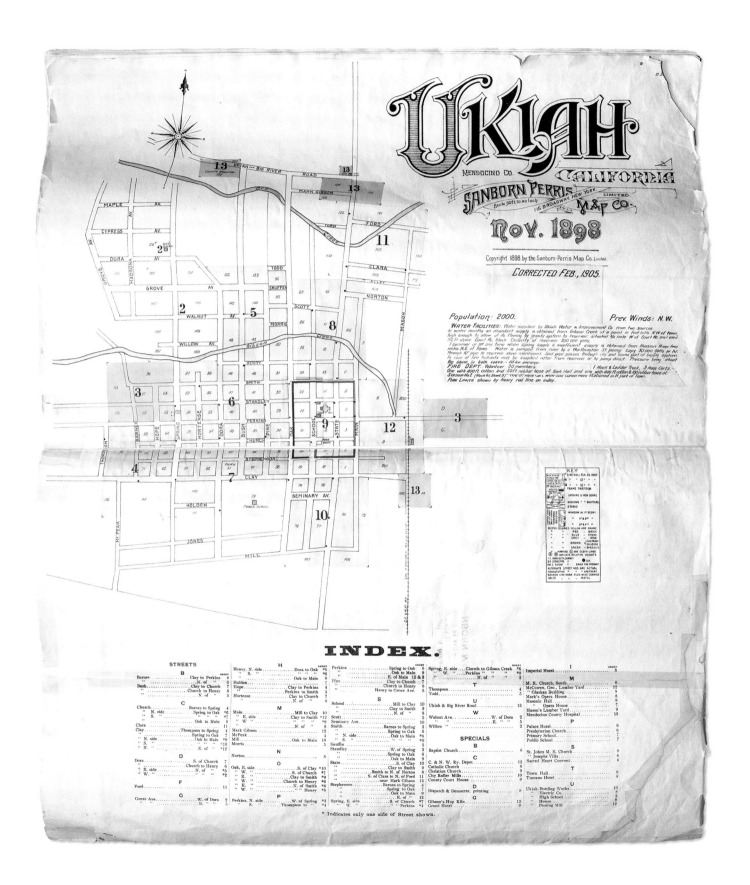

UKIAH

MENDOCINO CO. — CALIFORNIA

SANBORN-PERRIS MAP CO. LIMITED
115 BROADWAY, NEW YORK.
Scale 50 ft. to an inch.

Nov. 1898

Copyright 1898 by the Sanborn-Perris Map Co., Limited.

CORRECTED FEB., 1905.

Population: 2000.   Prev. Winds: N. W.

INDEX.

* Indicates only one side of Street shown.

Ukiah's Historically Significant Hospitals

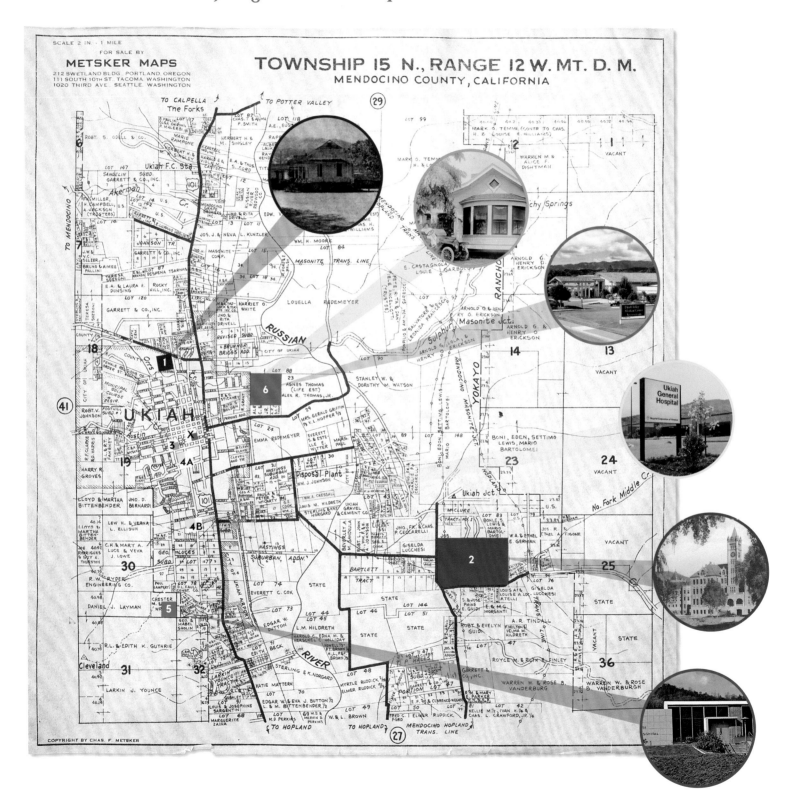

(Facing page)

1. Mendocino County Hospital & Farm
  Bush Street and Low Gap Road
  1881–1990 (last facility closed in 2001)
    1969: Renamed
    Mendocino Community Hospital
  Present: Mendocino County Planning Department;
  County Recorder; Juvenile Hall

2. Mendocino State Asylum for the Insane
  Talmage and Old River Roads, Talmage
  1889 Established; 1893–1972 Facility open
    1918: Renamed
    Mendocino State Hospital
  Present: City of 10,000 Buddhas, Dharma Realm
  Buddhist Association

X. Lathrop Hospital (not pictured)
  204 South Oak Street
  1902–1917: The practice of Dr. Ida May Lathrop-Malpus
  Present: Community Foundation of Mendocino County

3. Langland Hospital
  742 West Stephenson Street
  1913–1927: owned and operated by Cora Langland
  1927: Purchased by Theresa Ray for Ukiah General Hospital
  Present: Private home

4. Ukiah General Hospital
  1927–1957, Location 4A. 564 South Dora Street
  1957–1988, Location 4B. 1120 South Dora Street
    1972: Purchased by Hospital Corporation of America
    1976: New Facility completed
    1988: Closed

  Ukiah Adventist Hospital
  1988–2009, Location 4B. 1120 South Dora Street
    1988: Assets of Ukiah General purchased by Adventist Health
    1989: Renamed
    Ukiah Valley Medical Center
    Operated in tandem with Hospital Drive facility
  2009: South Dora Street facility sold
  to Mendocino County for use by Public Health
  Present: Mendocino County Health & Human Services

5. Hillside Community Hospital
  333 Laws Avenue
  1956–1980
    1966: Hillside becomes a non-profit
    1978: Purchased by Adventist Health
  1980: Moved to Hospital Drive facility and renamed
  Ukiah Adventist Hospital
  Present: Mendocino Community Health Clinic

6. Ukiah Adventist Hospital
  275 Hospital Drive
  1980–present
    1989: Renamed
    Ukiah Valley Medical Center
    1989–2009: Operated in tandem with South Dora Street facility
    2009: South Dora Street operations moved to Hospital Drive

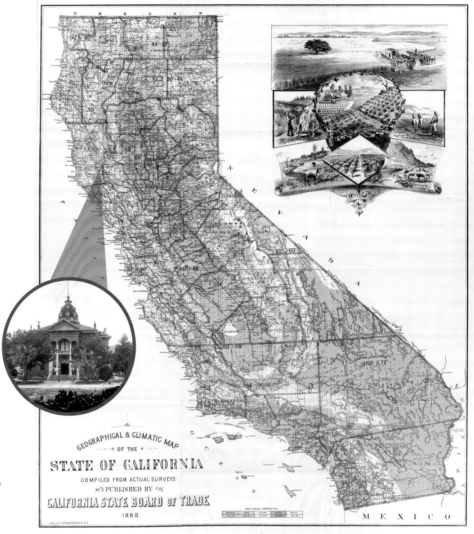

The city of Ukiah, located in northern California's Mendocino County, was founded in 1856 and became the county seat in 1859. The historic county courthouse pictured above was completed in 1873.

PREFACE

As the mother of a cancer-survivor, I owe my happiness to modern medicine and those who've dedicated their lives to it.

When my son, Grant, was sixteen months old, he was diagnosed with neuro blastoma, a childhood cancer with a terrifying mortality rate. I was seven months pregnant with my younger son, Sean, at the time. From March 2001 to March 2002, my husband, Justin, and I spent hours walking the halls of the University of California, San Francisco Medical Center (UCSF), wondering what lie ahead, always hoping for the best but knowing our baby's life depended on medical professionals who had a formidable challenge before them. For Grant to live, the medical team would have to remove the cancer wrapped around his spinal cord and invading his left thoracic cavity, compressing his left lung so no air could pass through it. After chemotherapy and several surgeries, Grant was pronounced cancer-free and every day since then has been a gift.

This book is one of the ways I hope to honor and appreciate the dedicated men and women of health care, the ones who dig for answers when they won't come easily, the ones who refuse to disconnect emotionally even though it would make life so much easier, the ones who put their patients before themselves day after day, night after night.

Thank you. I am profoundly grateful.

Jendi Coursey

ACKNOWLEDGMENTS

To be honest, this is the part of books I've always skipped. Now that I realize how much teamwork goes into writing a book, I have a new appreciation of the information conveyed in an acknowledgment.

My heartfelt thanks to Ukiah Valley Medical Center President Gwen Matthews and her husband Sam Ocampo who were inspired to capture the history of health care in Ukiah over dinner at Stars Restaurant in Ukiah. Sam read a little blurb about the history of the restaurant on the menu and asked Gwen if anyone had ever captured the story of health care in Ukiah. This book is the result.

I am incredibly grateful to the following talented, persistent, and thoughtful contributors without whom this book would not exist: researchers Lisa Ray and Julie Fetherston; photographer Evan Johnson; Theresa Whitehill, Adrienne Simpson, and Lillian Rubie of Colored Horse Studios; Ron Parker, Dr. Paul Poulos, and Barbara Webster from the Held-Poage Memorial Home and Research Library; Ukiah historian Ed Bold; Karen Holmes and Sherrie Smith-Ferri, PhD, from the Grace Hudson Museum; and several staff members from both Ukiah Valley Medical Center and the Mendocino County Health & Human Services Agency.

Thanks, also, to the people who spent hours sharing their stories: Earl Aagaard; Tamara Adams; Tom Allman; Mark Apfel, MD; Linda Ayotte, RD; Eula Barber; Nancy Biggins, Esq.; Dorothy Bowens, RN; Carolyn & Larry Brown; Robert Calson, MD; Jerry Chaney, RN; the Cleland family; Donald Coursey, MD; Karen Crabtree, MD; Phyllis Curtis; Dennis Denny; Phyllis Dockins, Mimi Doohan, MD; Susan Era; Charlie Evans, MD; Larry Falk, MD; Ron Gester, MD; Candy Gorbenko, RN; Herschel Gordon, MD; Brenda Hoek, RN; Kenneth Hoek, MD; Betty Hook; Lin Hunter; Ann Johnson, RN; Peter Keegan, MD; Maiga Lapkass; Marty Lombardi; Karena Massengill; Lynn Meadows, PA; Bill Mergener; Carol Mordhorst; Dale Morrison, MD; Wynd Nvotny; Sandy O'Ferrall; Noel O'Neill; Susan Pollesel, Ccc-Sp; Richard Roberts, MD; Barbara and Don Rones; Catherine Rosoff; Dick Selzer; Marvin Trotter, MD; Vince Valente, MD; the Vest family; Bill Waring, MD; Robert Werra, MD; Nyota Wiles, RN; Jacque Williams; Jim Withers, MD, PhD; and more.

Jendi Coursey

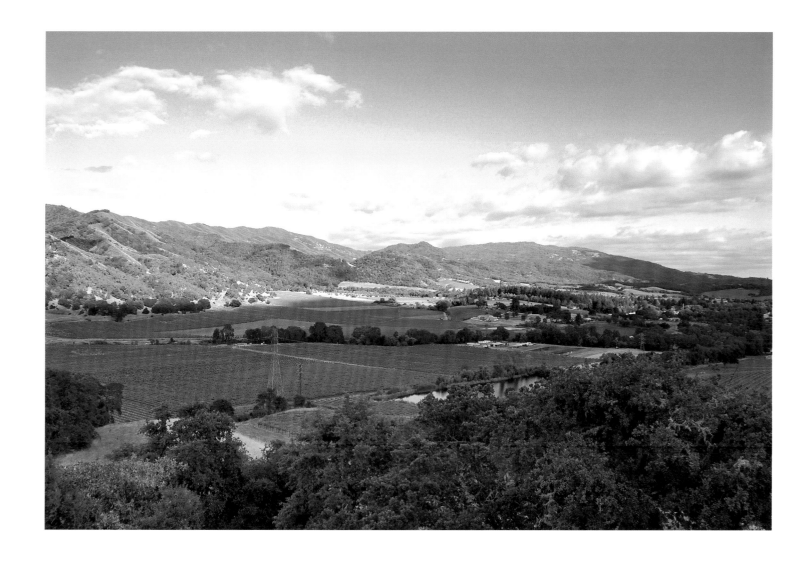

This book is dedicated to the men and women of health care,
the ones who dig for answers when they won't come easily, the
ones who refuse to disconnect emotionally even though it would
make life so much easier, the ones who put their patients before
themselves day after day, night after night.

FOREWORD

After my arrival in Ukiah, it did not take me long to realize that this was a very special place. Through the intriguing diversity of its people, there ran strong threads of shared values. I found people willing to invest impressive effort into building community relationships, who together supported the disadvantaged and downtrodden. It seemed to me that many Ukiahans demonstrated a great willingness to do whatever it took to make a difference.

Local people shared pieces of Ukiah's history with me. I heard stories of what had happened when people divided over differences as well as stories of incredible accomplishments when people came together. As someone who hoped to foster collaborative accomplishments, I was reminded of author Wes Adamson's quote: "Find something that you are passionate about in making a difference and you'll find a waiting kinship of people willing to unite for the cause." The more I learned about health care in Ukiah, the more convinced I became that great things could happen here.

When I began investigating the roots of health care in this community, I discovered that 2016 would mark the sixtieth anniversary of Ukiah Valley Medical Center's work here. What a great opportunity to capture and celebrate the stories of Ukiah's health care pioneers as well as record the circuitous route this town took to arrive where it is today with regard to health care.

Ukiah's health care professionals have risen to the challenges of an ever-changing landscape shaped by federal laws and funding, socioeconomic influences, and the winds of social change. Celebrating their work on behalf of the community was long overdue, and thus began the work of Jendi Coursey, whom we commissioned to capture this history of health care through those who experienced it and their descendants.

I invite you to delve into the pages of this book to meet this cast of colorful characters who, through their skill, knowledge, wit, and humor, left their mark on the lives of those they served.

Gwen Matthews, RN, MSc, MBA
President and CEO, Ukiah Valley Medical Center

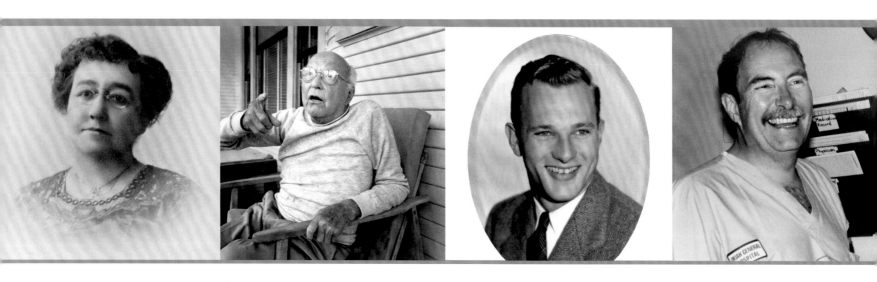

The city of Ukiah has always drawn a special breed of medical practitioner—people with the confidence and independence to work in a rural environment and the willingness to embrace a broad medical practice....

Ukiahness

AN INTRODUCTION

It takes a special kind of person to practice medicine in a small, rural town hours from the nearest big city. Unlike in the city, the support of colleagues and technology are not instantly available in small towns. The city of Ukiah, founded in 1856 and appointed the Mendocino County seat in 1859, has always drawn a special breed of medical practitioner—people with the confidence and independence to work in a rural environment and the willingness to embrace a broad medical practice, handling everything from earaches to wounds caused by an angry bull.

Ukiah is a typical American small town. People know their neighbors, and much to the chagrin of local teenagers, anonymity is rare. It takes about ten minutes to go from the north end of town to the south end if you hit all the red lights on State Street. In 2016 Ukiah had one movie theater, one bowling alley, one daily newspaper, and one main high school: Ukiah High, home of the Wildcats.

Located approximately 120 miles north of San Francisco on the Highway 101 corridor, the city of Ukiah covers almost five square miles in a valley surrounded by vineyards, pear orchards, and redwoods. The weather is temperate, and the area's natural beauty and clean air have always attracted people who enjoy the outdoors and who want a slower pace of life.

In fact in some ways, little has changed since Ukiah's *Dispatch Democrat* newspaper published an article on February 7, 1902, highlighting Dr. W. N. Moore's Ukiah Hospital and Sanitarium, stating, "This Sanitarium will doubtless grow rapidly in popularity, as Ukiah is an ideal location for such an institution. The purity of the air and the genial and equable climatic conditions are unsurpassed in the State."

Originally inhabited by Pomo peoples, the land that became the city of Ukiah was part of the Mexican land grant "Rancho Yokaya"

Opposite Left: Dr. Ida May Lathrop-Malpus began her practice in Ukiah in the early 1900s, and specialized in caring for women and children.

Opposite Center Left: Dr. Nicholas Zbitnoff served as a general practitioner in Ukiah for more than forty-four years, until his retirement in 1985.

Opposite Center Right: Dr. Hugh Curtis was one of Ukiah's first physicians to specialize in surgery; he served as a model physician in the community for thirty-six years.

Opposite Right: Dr. Laurence Hartley practiced as an obstetrician and gynecologist in Ukiah beginning in 1979. While he gave up his obstetrical practice in 2002, he continues to practice gynecology in 2016.

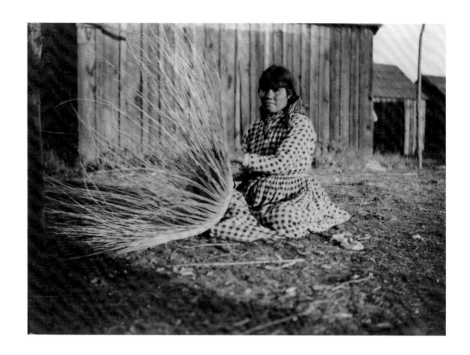

Right: Jenny Jackson weaves a twined basket at the Pinoleville Rancheria, 1892. Pomo baskets are widely admired as being among the finest in the world. Jackson was know for her weaving skill.

Below: Pickers at a hop camp, circa 1911.

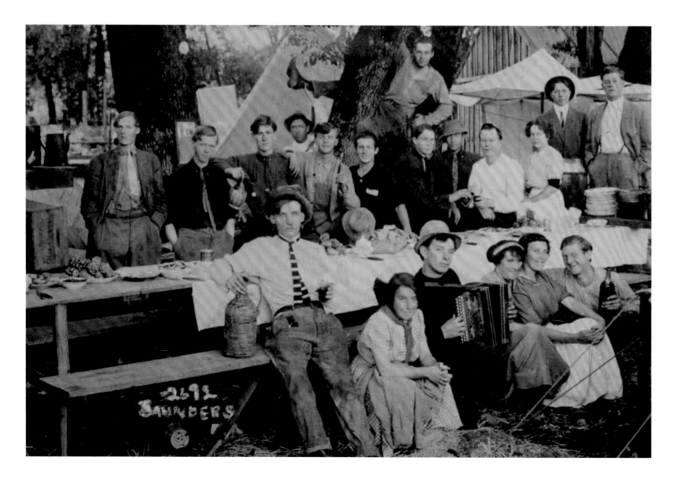

given by Alta California's Governor Pío Pico to Cayetano Juárez in 1845. The name *Ukiah* is an anglicized version of *Yokaya*, a Central Pomo word meaning "deep valley."

In 1889 the San Francisco Railroad and North Pacific Railroad connected Ukiah to the national rail network, making Ukiah more accessible and thus encouraging growth. Ukiah's population increased from about 1,850 in 1900 to 6,000 in 1950, then to 16,000 in 2010. The economic base has remained tied to the land through agriculture and lumber—from hops and redwoods to grapes and pears—as well as an influential illegal crop: marijuana. It is a town with a legacy from a bygone lumber industry coupled with a back-to-the-land movement, blending ranchers and hippies who have intermingled and intermarried, creating families and friendships with dramatic political and social diversity.

Since the city's founding, one of the most important traits that makes Ukiahans who they are is their willingness to take care of each other, whether in health care or in the broader community. When a need arises, people band together to fix a problem, fill a gap, or help a neighbor. While not unique to Ukiah, the idea of a small town taking care of its own has a special flavor in this Northern California locale. Mendocino County Sheriff Tom Allman said, "I don't know of any other communities where I've seen so many advertisements thanking the hospital for the care they've given, and not every community has a volunteer AIDS network."

Ukiah's size can make problems hard to ignore: homeless people are not hidden in the shadows, but seated on the grassy knolls around WalMart's parking lot. So while the town may be small, its challenges often are not. Ukiah's size can, however, make problems feel more manageable. Time and again, as Ukiah has faced problems common to the global community—such as hunger, cancer, AIDS, domestic violence, and homelessness—it has tackled each one and managed to care for local people. It has created humanitarian organizations such as Plowshares to feed the hungry; Cancer Resource Centers of Mendocino County to provide free support for cancer

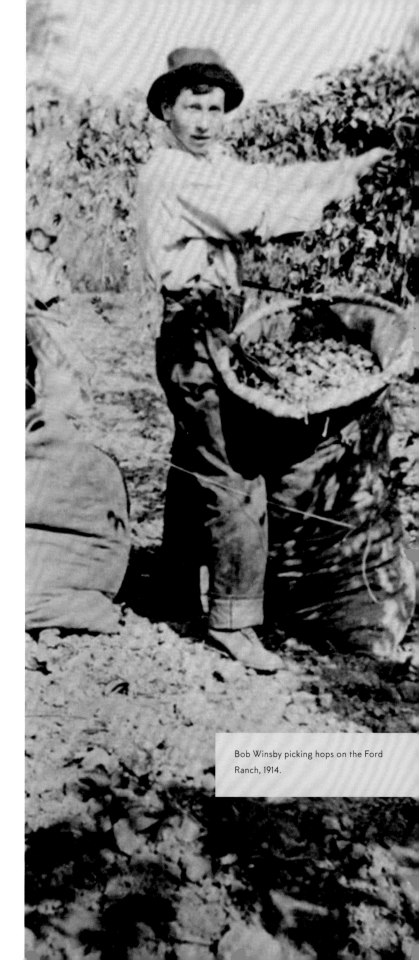

Bob Winsby picking hops on the Ford Ranch, 1914.

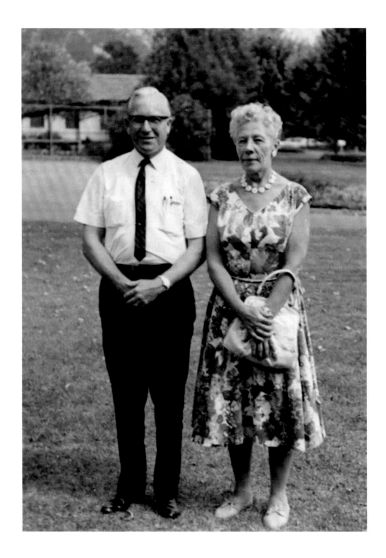

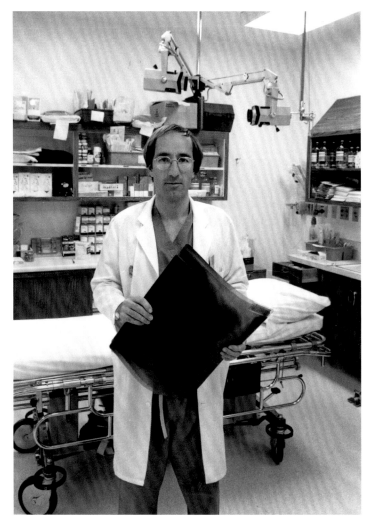

Left: John Brakebill and Dr. Louise E. Petty, Mendocino State Hospital, 1965.

Right: Dr. Ronald Gester, shown here in the Ukiah Valley Medical Center Emergency Department. He was instrumental in founding the Pacific Redwood Medical Group in 1993.

It just may be that Ukiah, with its small-town, I-can-do-it-myself attitude, can serve as a model to help national leaders view health care from a fresh perspective....

patients, Mendocino County AIDS/Viral Hepatitis Network to help patients navigate medical and social challenges associated with their diseases, Project Sanctuary to aid victims of domestic violence, and the Buddy Eller Center to support those suffering from addiction, among others. Small communities often support the development of relationships, and great things happen when people know and believe in each other.

As health care in the United States has grown increasingly complex and expensive, local hospitals and health care providers have expanded to meet the demand, found ways to finance state-of-the-art technology, and doggedly held to the notion that Ukiah can provide world-class care without being located in a big metropolitan area. The sentiment is, "We don't do everything, but what we do, we do well." While you may not find a specialty as narrow as pediatric neurosurgery because, thankfully, there just are not enough patients to support that type of practice, Ukiah's general surgeons are as good as or better than those you can find anywhere. And as Ukiahans look to the future of health care and see the impending crisis with the nationwide shortage of primary care doctors, they are working to bring a family medicine residency program to the area in the hope that educating doctors locally will provide a continual source of primary care physicians for local people.

It may just be that Ukiah, with its small-town, I-can-do-it-myself attitude, can serve as a model, helping national leaders recognize the importance of addressing health care issues community by community. Big-city solutions often depend on infrastructure that does not exist in rural locations, but this does not mean solutions do not exist for small towns. Maybe Ukiah can serve as a pebble with far-reaching ripples in the national health care pond.

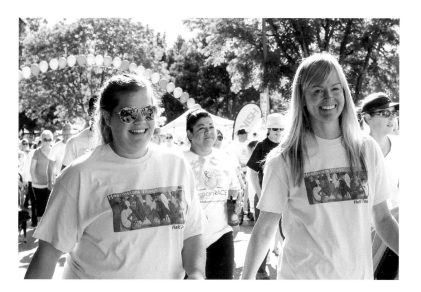

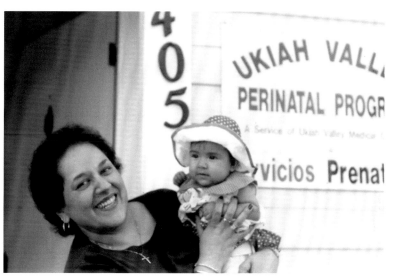

Top: Rachel Traywick and registered nurse Amy Warmerdam raise money for Hearthstone Village to support an orphanage in Haiti during Ukiah's annual Human Race fundraiser in 2014.

Bottom: Affectionately called the Greenhouse, Ukiah Valley Medical Center's Perinatal Program was housed in a light green house adjacent to the hospital at 1120 South Dora Street (originally the doctors' sleep house).

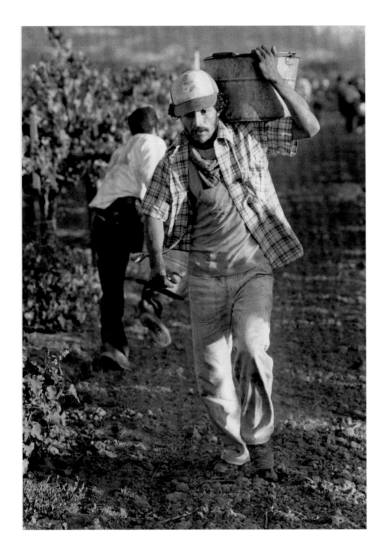

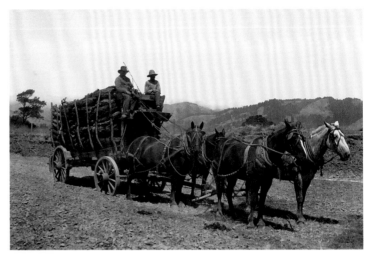

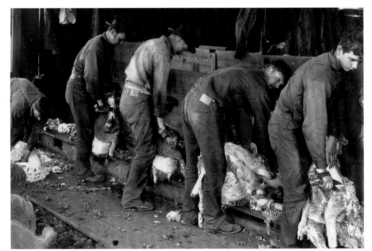

Above Left: Grape harvest in early fall.

Top Right: Two men with a wagonload of tanoak bark in Anderson Valley, 20 miles west of Ukiah.

Bottom Right: Men shearing sheep at the turn of the century.

The economic base has remained tied to the land through agriculture and lumber—from hops and redwoods to grapes and pears—as well as an influential illegal crop: marijuana.

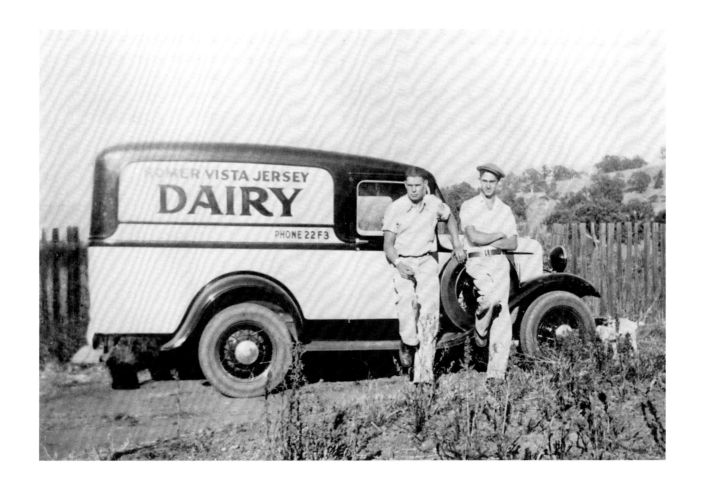

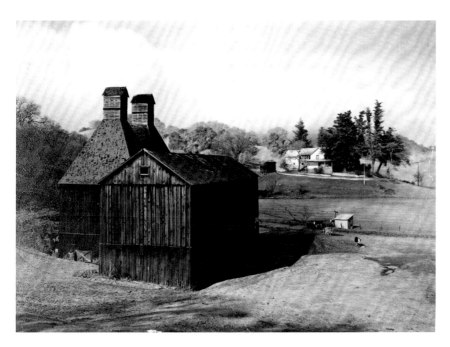

Above: Howard and Don Atkinson in front of the Romer Vista Jersey Dairy delivery truck #4 in the 1930s.

Left: Hop kiln at the old McGlashan Ranch, circa 1955.

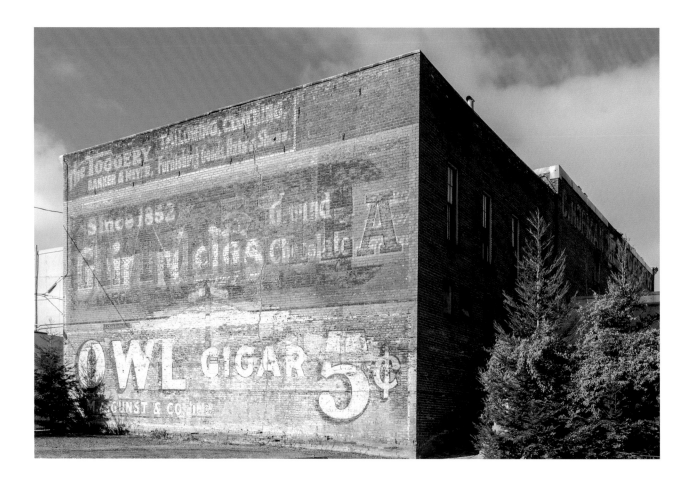

Above: Located on the corner of State and Standley Streets, the McKinley building has housed local businesses since it was built in 1908, beginning with the Ukiah Post Office.

Right: A rainbow over vineyards adjacent to Redemeyer Road in the Ukiah valley after a fall shower.

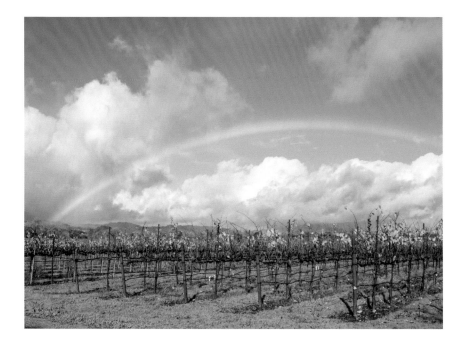

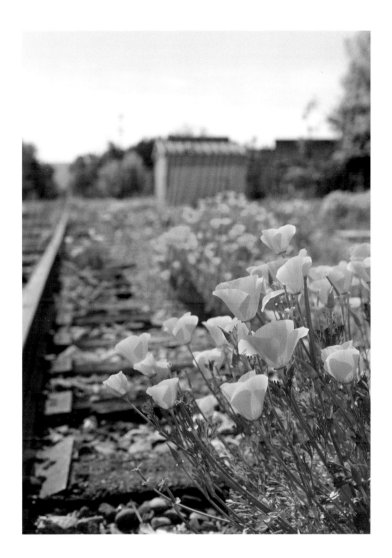

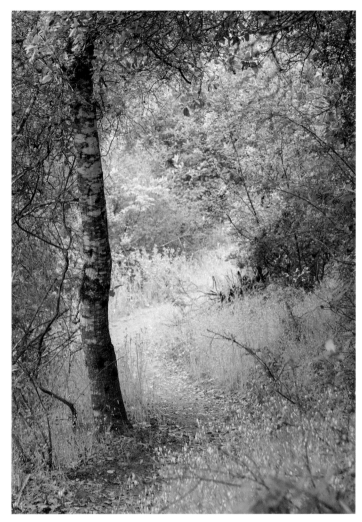

"Ukiah is an ideal location for such an institution [the Ukiah Hospital and Sanitarium]. The purity of the air and the genial and equable climatic conditions are unsurpassed in the State."

–Ukiah Dispatch Democrat, *1902*

Left: Spring poppies grow along the abandoned railroad tracks near Perkins Street, not far from downtown Ukiah.

Right: A winding path in Low Gap Park on the west side of Ukiah.

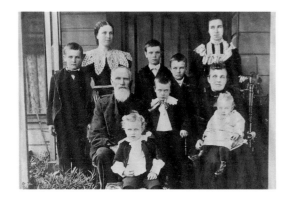

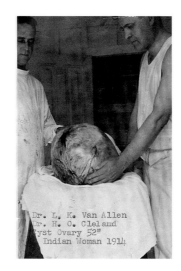

Dr. L. K. Van Allen
Dr. H. O. Cleland
Cyst Ovary 52"
Indian Woman 1914

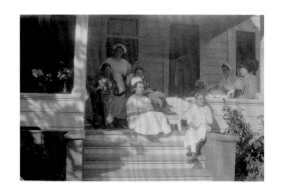

Hillside
Community
Hospital

Hospital closed

Lathrop Hospital

Purchased by Ukiah
General Hospital

Ukiah founded

Langland Hospital   Ukiah General Hospital

1856

1889

1902   1913 1917

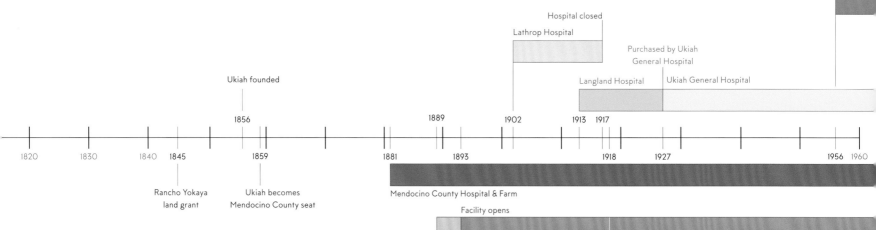

1820   1830   1840   1845   1859   1881   1893   1918   1927   1956 1960

Rancho Yokaya
land grant

Ukiah becomes
Mendocino County seat

Mendocino County Hospital & Farm

Facility opens

Mendocino State Asylum for the Insane   Renamed
Mendocino State Hospital

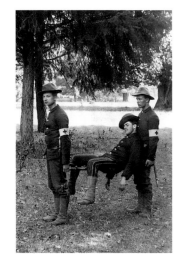

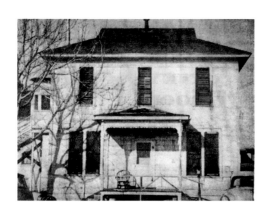

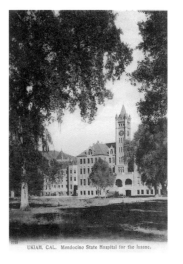

UKIAH, CAL. Mendocino State Hospital for the Insane.

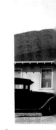

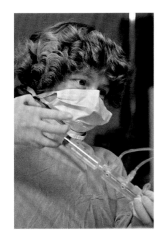

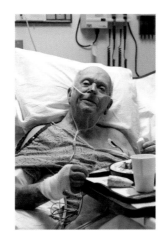

Our Hospitals

BUILDING BLOCKS OF UKIAH'S
MODERN HEALTH CARE

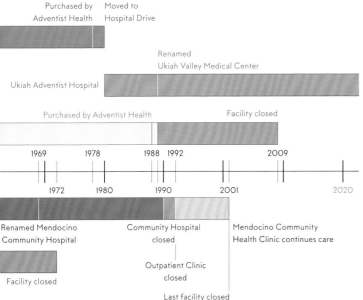

Purchased by Adventist Health Moved to Hospital Drive

Renamed Ukiah Valley Medical Center

Ukiah Adventist Hospital

Purchased by Adventist Health Facility closed

1969   1978   1988 1992   2009

1972   1980   1990   2001   2020

Renamed Mendocino Community Hospital Community Hospital closed Mendocino Community Health Clinic continues care

Outpatient Clinic closed

Facility closed

Last facility closed

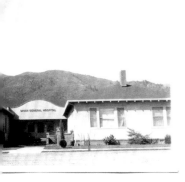

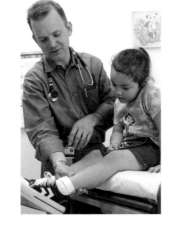

Historically, people received all their health care at home. The earliest medical practitioners in Ukiah, the native Pomo peoples, used prayer, spiritual dances, herbs, and poultices to heal their sick and wounded. When non-native settlers came into the valley, primarily from the Midwest, they also cared for one another at home—first out of necessity, then out of choice.

Although hospitals had become more commonplace by the early 1900s, people still birthed babies at home and doctors made house calls to treat most medical problems; unless surgery was called for, those who could afford to stay out of hospitals did so. The term *hospital* covered a wide range of facilities, from a room in someone's home to large structures built specifically to house and care for the sick. In many communities, at least one hospital doubled as a poorhouse, separating the undesirables—the poor, elderly, orphaned, contagious, and mentally ill—from the rest of the community, and Ukiah was no exception. And although people went to hospitals to receive care, until twentieth-century breakthroughs in sterilization, anesthesia, antisepsis, and antibiotics, doctors had very few tools with which to aid their patients; in many people's minds, hospitals were where the sick went to die. But hospitals evolved as technology and pharmacology advanced, and by the mid-1950s the foundation for Ukiah's modern health care delivery system was firmly established. People went in sick and often came out substantially healed.

All history starts somewhere, and the beginning of modern American medicine in Ukiah began in the mid-1950s. The hospitals described on the following pages existed in Ukiah in the 1950s, but their histories go back decades before. Each hospital's story

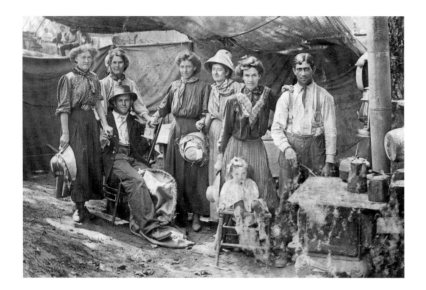

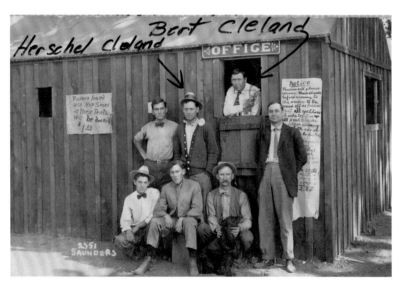

starts when the hospital first opened, beginning with the two public hospitals: Mendocino County Hospital and Farm, which opened in 1881; and the Mendocino State Asylum for the Insane, which was established in 1889 and opened in 1893. While some private hospitals opened and closed in the decades that followed, the only private hospitals treating patients in the 1950s were Ukiah General Hospital, which began as Langland Hospital in 1913 and Hillside Community Hospital (later Ukiah Valley Medical Center), which opened in 1956.

These facilities, and the care provided therein, were typical for their eras. The hospitals grew or changed based on community needs and available funding. They followed health care's evolution from generalized to specialized medicine, from high-touch (relationship-based) care to high tech treatment, and eventually found a blend to incorporate the best of both approaches.

Top: A family makes camp during hop-picking season in the early 1900s.

Bottom: H. O. Cleland and Bert Cleland pose for a photo with others at the ranch office where hop pickers were paid. Note the sign that reads, "Pickers found with hop socks in their tents will be docked $1.00."

MENDOCINO COUNTY HOSPITAL AND FARM—CARING FOR THE POOR

The County Hospital and Farm opened in 1881 as a residential hospital dedicated to serving the poor. According to newspaper articles of the time, the 155-acre property north of town was originally "Tom Gibson's place" and included a farm, garden, and dairy herd. Located on the southwest corner of Bush Street and Low Gap Road, the hospital was built for $4,000 and attending physician Dr. W. N. Moore ministered to about sixty patients when the facility opened.

E. W. Mankins served as steward, managing the business side of the operation—no small task given that once patients recovered from their medical conditions, they often remained at the farm, living in small cabins and working to repay the cost of their care, room, and board. Admissions records from 1892 indicate that most of the patients were men with no property and no health insurance, and many remained at the facility for the rest of their lives. The county hospital facility went on to serve the community for more than seventy years with just a few changes to the structure, including a $1,000 tuberculosis ward built in 1917.

While larger metropolitan areas began to separate their sick from their needy, Mendocino County continued to use the County Hospital and Farm as a catchall for indigents and even inmates. In the 1930s, county physician Dr. Herschel Orville "H. O." Cleland was deputized, so the sheriff's office could send petty criminals and public inebriates to County Farm to work off their sentences.

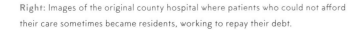

Right: Images of the original county hospital where patients who could not afford their care sometimes became residents, working to repay their debt.

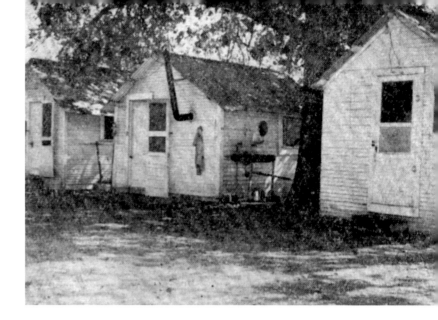

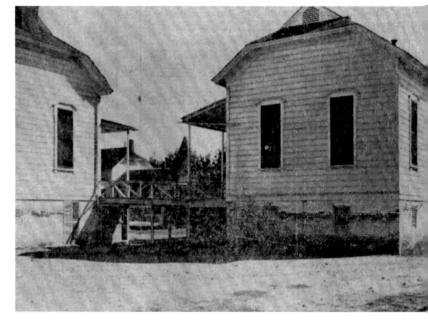

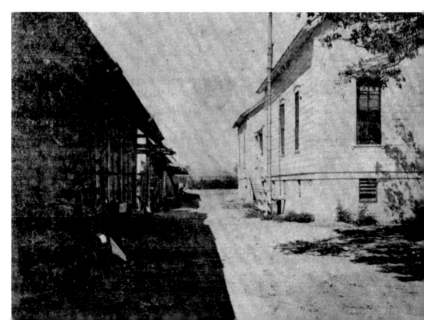

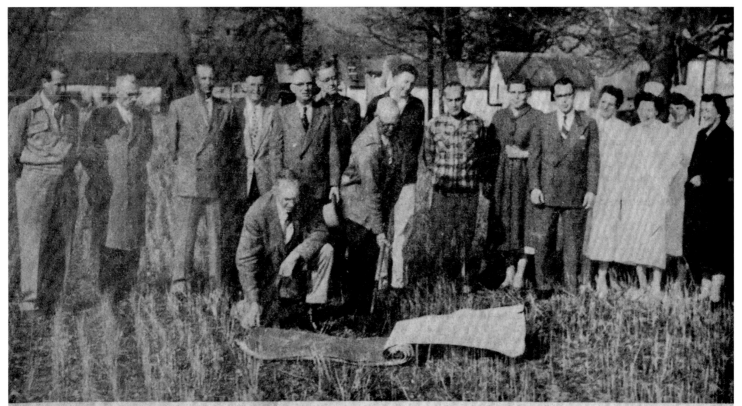

GROUND BREAKING CEREMONIES for the million dollar Mendocino county hospital took place this morning, with Former Supervisor George Decker wielding the shovel. Decker was on the board when much of the work preparatory to obtaining federal and state aid for the project took place. Kneeling beside Decker is Supervisor Joseph Hartley. Standing, left to right, are E. Aadland, superintendent of construction for Utah Construction Company of San Francisco, which has the contract for erecting the 83-bed hospital; V. O. Tyler and T. C. Tillman, also Utah Construction Company officials; Supervisors Joseph Scaramella and Harold Bainbridge; Dr. C. R. Kroeger, director of the Mendocino county health department; Claude Falconer, president of the Ukiah Chamber of Commerce; Bert Mankins, county hospital superintendent; Margaret Bernard, public health nurse for the county; Dr. John O. Raffety, medical director at the county hospital; and Vera Snider, Betty Glynn, Dorothy Bowen and Shirley Lilienthal, county hospital nurses. Chairman Paul Poulos of the board of supervisors is vacationing in Mexico and so unable to be present.   JOURNAL photo by Cober

The updated facility was touted as a modern eighty-three-bed hospital offering an isolated fourteen-bed tuberculosis wing, thirty-six acute-care beds, twenty-two beds for the chronically ill, and three psychiatric beds. It included a separate outpatient clinic, two surgery rooms, a delivery room, maternity and pediatric wards, and a lead-lined X-ray room. The kitchen was described as a "modern marvel of stainless steel."

By the 1950s the buildings were in desperate need of renovation, so county supervisors took advantage of funding through the Hill-Burton Act to rebuild. The Act offered a three-way match with federal, state, and county funds, and those funds came with a twenty-year mandate requiring the hospital to accept all patients, regardless of their ability to pay, and to provide a certain percentage of care completely free of cost. As this had been the facility's purpose since its inception, caring for the poor did not feel like an insurmountable burden. Affording this care, however, became increasingly difficult.

The updated facility was touted as a modern eighty-three-bed hospital offering an isolated fourteen-bed tuberculosis wing, thirty-six acute-care beds, twenty-two beds for the chronically ill, and three psychiatric beds. It included a separate outpatient clinic, two surgery rooms, a delivery room, maternity and pediatric wards, and a lead-lined X-ray room. The kitchen was described as a "modern marvel of stainless steel, giant electric mixers, and meat saws." The renovated hospital opened on January 21, 1957, and for the next decade, it provided care to indigent patients throughout the county.

Things changed dramatically in the 1960s when Congress approved federal health care funding in the form of Medicare and Medicaid, and California adopted Medi-Cal. Indigent patients now had a choice about where to receive care, and they often chose the local private hospitals: Ukiah General Hospital and Hillside Community Hospital. Private doctors who had not been invited to practice at County Hospital declined to bring indigent patients there now that federal funding was available at their preferred hospitals. Doctors who practiced at General and Hillside felt the county facility was subpar.

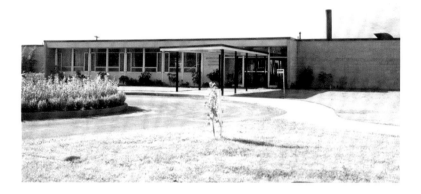

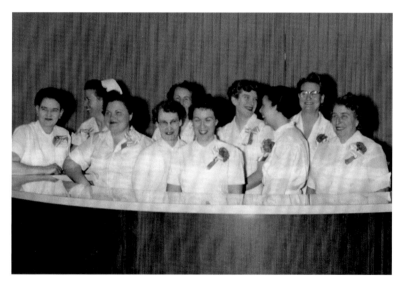

Above: In 1957, the new county hospital was completed. In 2016, county offices remain at corner of Bush and Low Gap Streets.

Below: Nurses from County Hospital celebrate opening day in 1957.

Opposite: Mendocino County supervisors join members of the Mendocino County Hospital staff at the ground-breaking ceremony for the new county hospital, which was located on Dora Street in Ukiah.

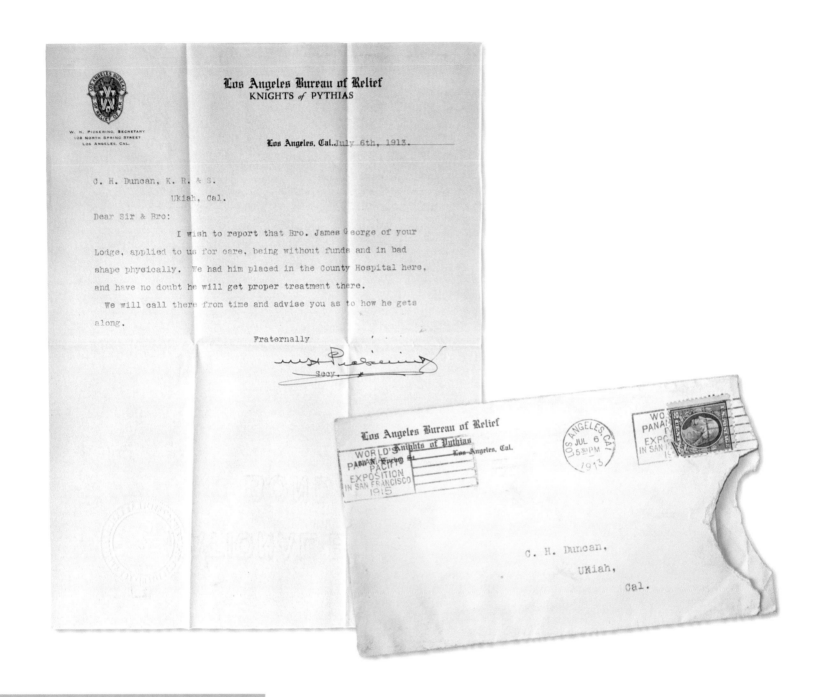

Like other county hospitals of its time, the Mendocino County Hospital and Farm cared for the most disenfranchised people in the community for decades.

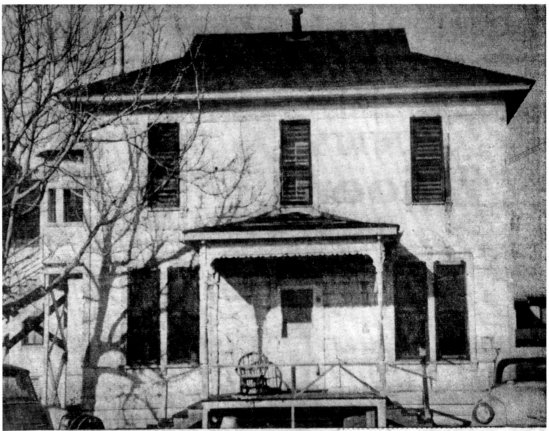

OUTLASTED ITS USEFULNESS—This is Ward 6, Mendocino County Hospital, which is soon to give way to the march of progress and has been offered for sale for $74, with several takers. One of the original buildings of the hospital, it is the only 2-story structure and is located at the south end of the grounds, a good example of the type of construction half a century ago. The hospital grounds were owned before the hospital was begun by Thomas Jefferson Gibson, grandfather of Judge Lilburn Gibson, and provided him with some favorite hunting in that early day.

JOURNAL photo by Cober

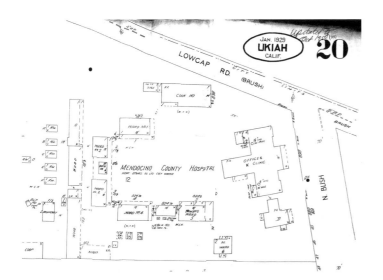

Above: Ward 6 of the Mendocino County Hospital, built in the 1880s, was offered for sale at seventy-four dollars in 1956.

Left: This map shows the layout of the Mendocino County Hospital as it was in 1929.

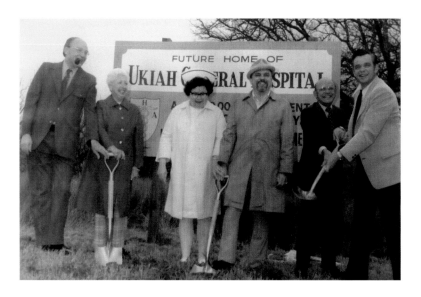

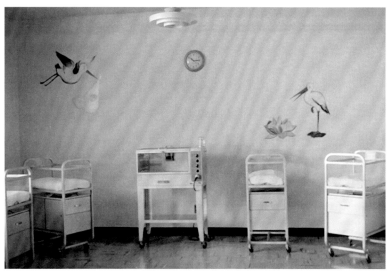

Top: While the county struggled to maintain hospital operations, Ukiah General Hospital broke ground on a new facility. The nurse in the center is head nurse Juanita Burke.

Bottom: Hillside Community Hospital opened in 1956 and cared for newborns in this nursery.

Mendocino Community Hospital

In 1969, the county hospital was renamed Mendocino Community Hospital (MCH), and the county began tracking hospital finances through an enterprise fund rather than bundling them in with the general fund. By 1972, it was clear that the cost of care for long-term, chronically ill patients outstripped state and federal reimbursement, so MCH closed long-term care beds and became a fifty-six-bed hospital.

Only about a third of MCH beds were regularly in use in 1979, yet between 1969 and 1979 taxpayers had invested approximately $1.6 million in the facility, which consistently operated at a substantial deficit.[1] The two private hospitals in Ukiah, Ukiah General and Hillside Community, ran at capacity or close to it, but could not expand because NorCoa, the region's state-appointed agency to regulate hospital beds and limit duplication of services, determined the Ukiah area could only support a combined total of 144 hospital beds.

The patients who did continue to seek county services were those in need of mental health care, but the void left by the closure of Mendocino State Hospital for the mentally ill in 1972 left county medical professionals overwhelmed with these patients, who had little money to pay for their care. By the late 1970s, the hospital's financial challenges led county supervisors to seek a way out of the hospital business; however, Mendocino Community Hospital supporters drafted and helped pass Proposition A, which discouraged county supervisors from shuttering the facility in the near term.

Even through financial hardship, MCH continued to care for the most disenfranchised people in the community, and the doctors who treated these patients were a breed apart, often

Ukiah Daily Journal

Thursday, December 6, 1979

Year No. 197   468-0123   Ukiah, Mendocino County, California   5 Sections   20 Cents

Inside

President Carter says he is prepared to begin putting pressure on Iran in order to win the release of hostages held at the American Embassy. See story, Page 3.

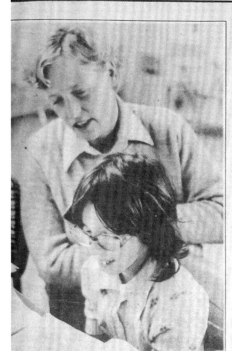

AN ASSIST WITH LEARNING
Tutor Barbara Johnson and Sandy Pryse, 11

Photo by Dale Kalkman

ollege students
toring Pomolita kids

By VICKY KEMP
Journal Staff Writer

Community Hospital

Should it be closed? Forum-goers find
the answer depends on who you ask

By MITCHELL LANDSBERG
Journal Staff Writer

Dr. Hugh Curtis accurately described it as a matter of perception.

The answer to the question of closing Mendocino Community Hospital, he said, depended on who was asked and what their experiences had been.

That seemed to be the case Wednesday evening as some 200 people jammed the Palace Hotel ballroom to hear Curtis and Dr. Phranklin Apfel gently debate the merits of keeping Community open.

In Curtis' view: "Community Hospital is not a viable, adequate institution in which we can practice quality medical care."

In Apfel's opinion: "There are many patients who find that the atmosphere at the Community Hospital is more conducive to their healing process."

With style often merging with substance, the two doctors tangled over the quality and profitability of health care at the county-owned hospital. Curtis is a surgeon and member of the Medical Society of Mendocino and Lake Counties, which has taken a strong position against keeping Community Hospital open. Apfel is chief of staff at Community, and the most outspoken advocate of retaining the hospital.

The hospital forum was sponsored by the Greater Ukiah Chamber of Commerce. Daily Journal publisher Jim Garner served as moderator.

While most of the discussion covered familiar ground for those acquainted with the hospital debate, Apfel opened up new territory with figures he said came from a county audit of Community Hospital which has not yet been released.

The audit, he said, showed that the hospital is close to being profitable.

And, Apfel argued, the closure of Community would cost the county a fortune in direct and indirect costs.

After a long and intricate analysis of the hospital's financial situation, Apfel concluded the county would lose a total of $3,300,000 annually if it closed Community.

And, he said, with proper management, Community could be making a profit of $200,000 to $500,000 a year.

(County Supervisor Norman deVall, a member of the supervisors' health and welfare committee, said today that the audit to which Apfel referred is not yet complete. "The audit is virtually completed," he said, "but not in the hands of the county." DeVall said the accounting firm hired for the audit has sent county officials "a rudimentary balance sheet," which he said shows a "bottom-line loss of about $71,000" annually at the hospital. But, he said, "I don't believe (Apfel) would have a full copy of the audit.")

Apfel said Community can save taxpayers money because its revenues go back into county coffers, while Hillside and General Hospital keep their profits. Apfel argued that all hospitals keep afloat through federal and state funding and Medicare payments, but in the case of Community, the government money goes back into public hands.

He said he thought Hillside and General "are interested in getting that $3,300,000 into their own (facilities)."

"Let's keep it here in our community hospital," he said.

Apfel said Community currently "covers 95 percent of its losses," and could cut out much of the expense that sent it into the red last year by canceling its contract with National Medical Enterprises, the hospital's hired out-of-town administrators.

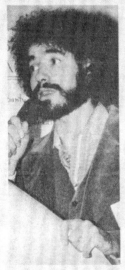

Dr. PHRANKLIN APFEL
Community Chief of staff

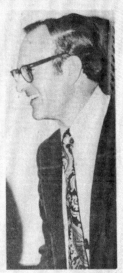

Dr. HUGH CURTIS
Representing Medical Society

Apfel said NME was providing "poor management," and said Community could do better with local administrators.

He said the hospital presently has reserves of $385,000.

"We're not losers," he said. "We have the most potential of any institution in the county to bring money into the county."

Curtis said Apfel "is the only one (Continued on Page 2)

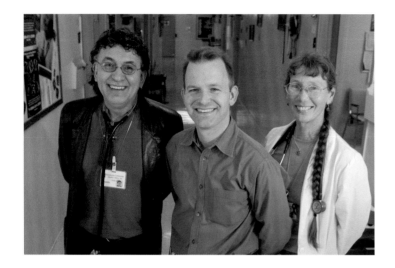

having more in common with the counterculture than the establishment. MCH medical staff members Dr. Phranklin Apfel and his cousin Dr. Mark Apfel had bushy beards and wore Birkenstocks and Hawaiian shirts. They were sometimes called the Smith Brothers after the cough drops featuring two similar figures. According to Dr. Mark Apfel, the most common reason for hospital admission at MCH was alcohol withdrawal, but doctors also treated many patients with infectious diseases, such as tuberculosis. Then, in the 1980s, Ukiah's proximity to San Francisco put it on the frontline of a terrifying new virus, the first retro-virus in America: acquired immune deficiency syndrome (AIDS). The first patients diagnosed with AIDS in Ukiah were diagnosed at Mendocino Community Hospital.

In the early 1990s, after years of financial instability, MCH closed the doors of its public hospital (in August 1990) and its outpatient clinic (in 1992); it closed its psychiatric facility in November 2001.

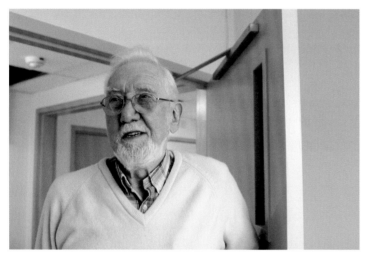

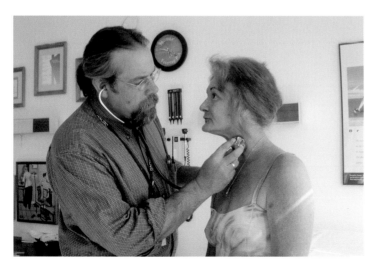

Top: Physician assistant Amunka Davila, pediatrician and internal medicine physician Dr. Jorge "JJ" Allende, and nurse practitioner Cottie Morrison provided outpatient care for Mendocino Community Health Clinic's Hillside Health Center.

Center: Dr. Bill Fisher worked as a thoracic surgeon in Ukiah. During his later years, he helped Mendocino Community Hospital's successor receive accreditation from the Joint Commission on the Accreditation of Healthcare.

Bottom: Physician assistant Thomas Feiertag has worked for Hillside Health Center since its inception.

Mendocino Community Health Clinic

In 1992, when the county stopped providing outpatient medical services, local clinics took patients in. In Ukiah, county supervisors helped facilitate a seamless transition for outpatient care through Mendocino Community Health Clinic (MCHC) by permitting MCHC to occupy the former county outpatient clinic building located on Bush Street. MCHC provided medical, dental, and behavioral health care. That same year Mendocino County was named a "Medically Underserved Population" (MUP) and a "Health Professionals Shortage Area" (HPSA); MCHC was certified as a "Federally Qualified Health Center" (FQHC) and was therefore allowed to bill Medicare and Medi-Cal for its services.

These designations helped pave the way for increased payments (higher than the usual rates), which attracted more clinical professionals to the region. Doctors and dentists who chose to practice at Mendocino Community Health Clinic and care for the underserved could qualify to have part of their medical or dental school debt forgiven.

Under the leadership of Linnea Ritter-Hunter, MCHC continued the tradition of caring for the community's most vulnerable and eventually moved into the building that originally housed Hillside Community Hospital. During the next twenty years, MCHC expanded to add health centers in Willits and Lakeport, which brought millions of dollars to the region through federal funding and capital grants and eventually allowed for the treatment of more than five hundred patients per day. Hunter continued to advocate for health care for the poor and underrepresented populations in Ukiah until her retirement in 2015, when MCHC's Chief Operations Officer Carole Press took over as chief executive officer.

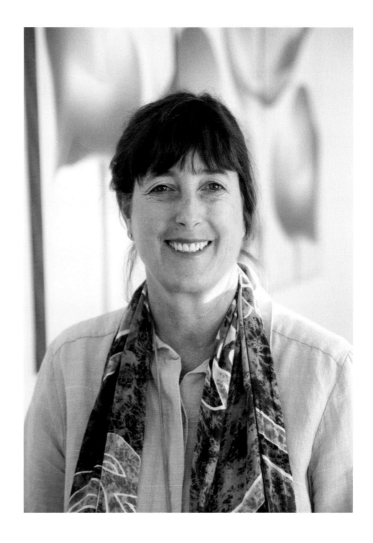

Obstetrician and gynecologist Dr. Karen Crabtree cared for vulnerable populations at home and abroad, treating women in Africa and on a Navajo Indian reservation. Since 2007, she has served as the medical director at Mendocino Community Health Clinic's women's health service, Care for Her.

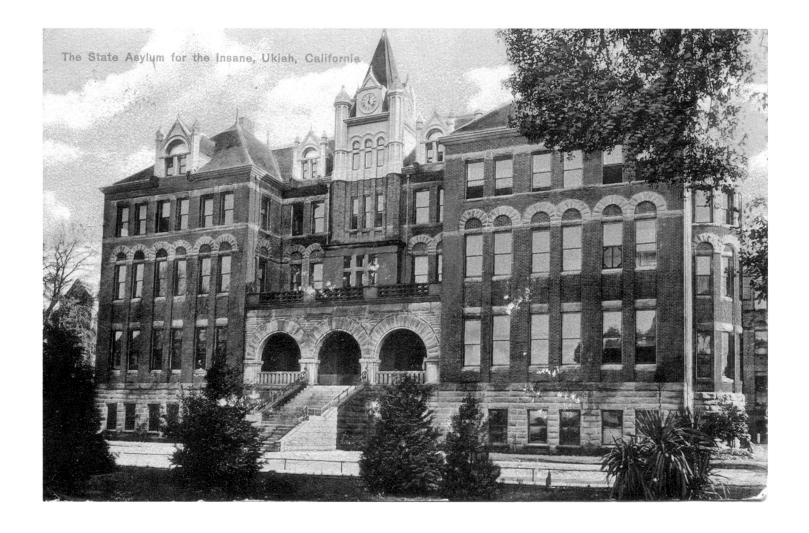

The State Asylum for the Insane, Ukiah, California

One of the state hospital's most profound effects on health care in Ukiah, in addition to the care it provided, was serving as a magnet for well-trained physician specialists who would otherwise never have come to the area.

MENDOCINO STATE ASYLUM
FOR THE INSANE

The history of mental health care in Ukiah—and throughout the United States—has been plagued by fear and ignorance. Before the 1800s, mentally ill family members were sometimes confined in "stronghouses," or cells on a family's property. If a family could not afford to house their mentally ill, the patient could be sold at auction and someone with enough means and the willingness to clothe, feed, and confine the person would take on the charge.[2] If a suitable home could not be found, the mentally ill were hospitalized in deplorable conditions in public poorhouses, often alongside criminals and the destitute. Private madhouses run by clergy were sometimes an option for more well-to-do families, but treatments—consisting of prayers, charms, and amulets to ward off evil spirits—were ineffective. Sedatives, including opium grains, were sometimes used to ease the patient's (or caregiver's) suffering but did not provide lasting improvement.

Through the decades, doctors dedicated to understanding and shining a light on the mysteries of the mind have helped patients and the greater community approach mental health with insight and compassion rather than fear and derision. Psychiatry was one of the first medical specialties, and as early as the 1880s, state lawmakers recognized mental health care as a public issue separate from medical care, having its own challenges and requiring its own resources. Thus began the institutionalization of psychiatric patients in California. The Mendocino State Asylum for the Insane was established in 1889 and opened its doors in Ukiah on December 12, 1893, with local psychiatrist Dr. Edward Warren King as superintendent.

The hospital was built in Talmage on one hundred acres purchased from the Bartlett brothers.[3] Upon opening, the asylum received 150 male patients from three state hospitals in Napa, Stockton, and Angus, filling the hospital immediately. One year later, a wing for females opened. Hospital buildings then separated patients based on gender and patient type (the noisy and hard-to-manage in one

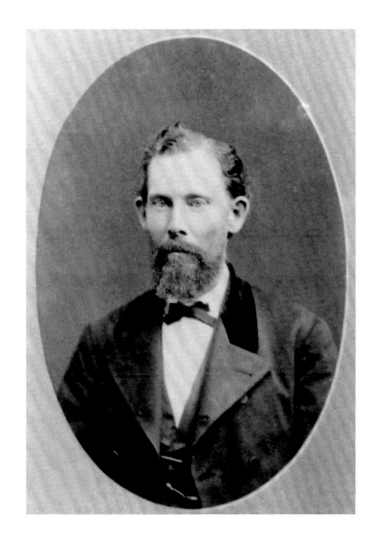

Superintendent of Mendocino State Asylum for the Insane Dr. E. W. King, circa 1895.

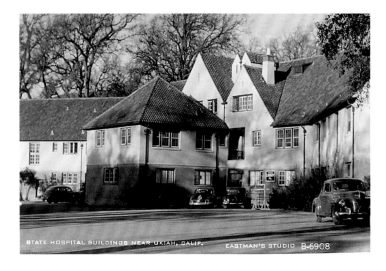

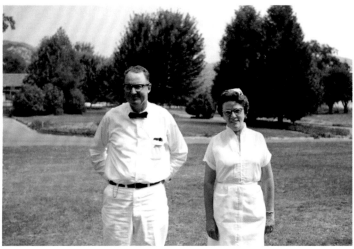

Top: Here is an old ward prior to being remodeled into the Receiving and Treatment building, circa 1950.

Bottom: Beecher F. Conover and Agnes Chapman at Mendocino State Hospital, 1966.

building, and the quiet and calm in another). In 1918, the state legislature renamed the facility Mendocino State Hospital. The patient population steadily grew, particularly after the stock market crash in 1929. In 1932, the hospital had more than 1,900 patients and three hundred staff members, representing almost two-thirds of Ukiah's entire population. The 1930 census indicates Ukiah's population was 3,124.

Mendocino State Hospital

In 1952, the original hospital building was demolished and new buildings were erected to address changing needs. The facility had become a city within a city with its own farm, bakery, and dairy herd, and it supported approximately 2,400 patients and eight hundred employees at a time when Ukiah's entire population was only 6,120.[4]

The hospital employed the last shoemaker to be paid by the State of California. After serving as a driver in the Ambulance Corps during World War I, Cherubino Valentini made shoes at Mendocino State Hospital for thirty-five years, from 1919 until his retirement in 1955.

Because the psychiatric patients were full-time residents, the hospital had to provide them with more than just psychiatric care; patients received medical and dental care, physical therapy, occupational therapy, and recreation, necessitating a medical staff capable of a broad spectrum of care. Eventually, specialty care included podiatry, urology, gynecology, orthopedics, otolaryngology (ear, nose, and throat), ophthalmology, and optometry; programs included medical and surgical care, psychiatric care, alcohol and drug rehabilitation, vocational training, a pharmacy, and treatment for the criminally insane (from 1929 to 1954). The hospital also sustained a psychiatric residency program and a student nurse program.

A Day in the Life

Former psychiatric technician Ron Parker said,

"We used to take the patients outside almost every day, weather permitting. Only 'good' patients—no escape risks, combative ones or ill folks. A typical day shift included wake up, dress after shower, medications (if needed), breakfast, and patient count on the ward. Then it was free time, out to the yard until lunch. After lunch, it was medications and back outside or into the day room to watch TV. Evenings were spent watching TV or off the ward to a movie or a dance one or two days a week. Now this was for the patients on the back wards and all patients prior to the early 1960s. After that, things changed. But this photo was from the old days."

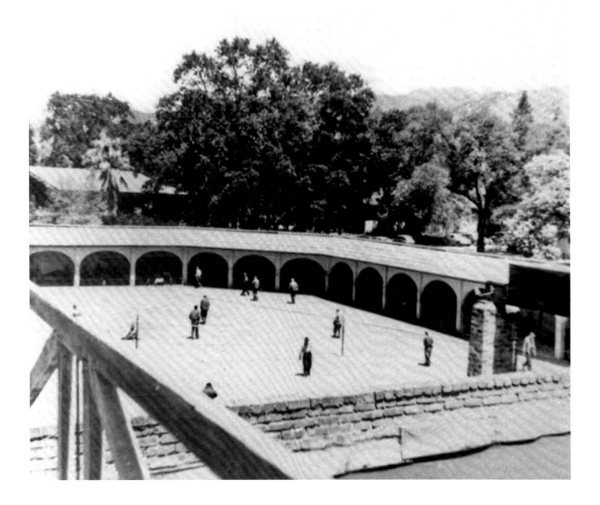

Patients who were not escape risks or combative often spent time in the open space inside the ward. This photo was taken prior to 1955.

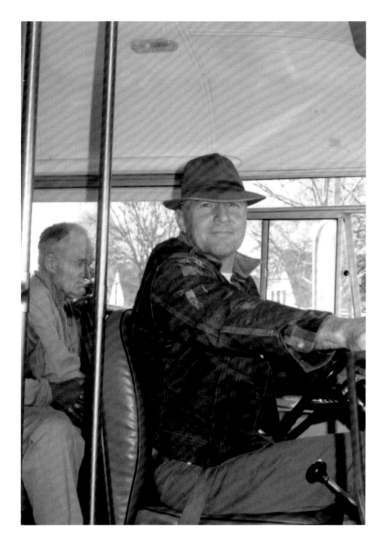

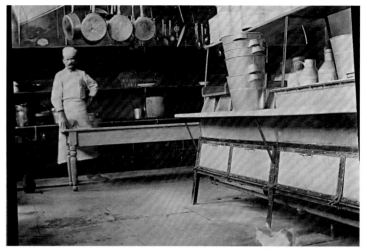

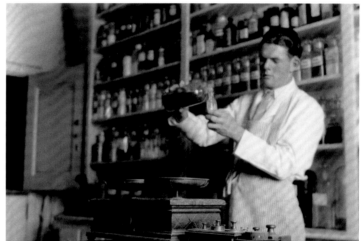

The Mendocino State Hospital (MSH) was a city within a city. The hospital purchased leather and made shoes. It purchased tin for the cannery, and filled the tins with fruits and vegetables from its gardens. Staff made clothes, raised hogs, ran a successful dairy, and sometimes patients boarded the MSH bus to go on outings like ballgames, picnics, or to see a movie. The hospital had its own apothecary and a huge kitchen.

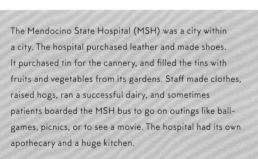

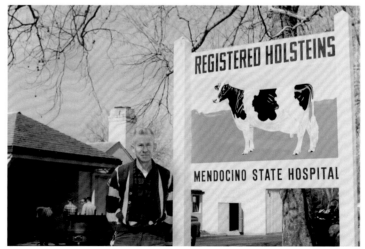

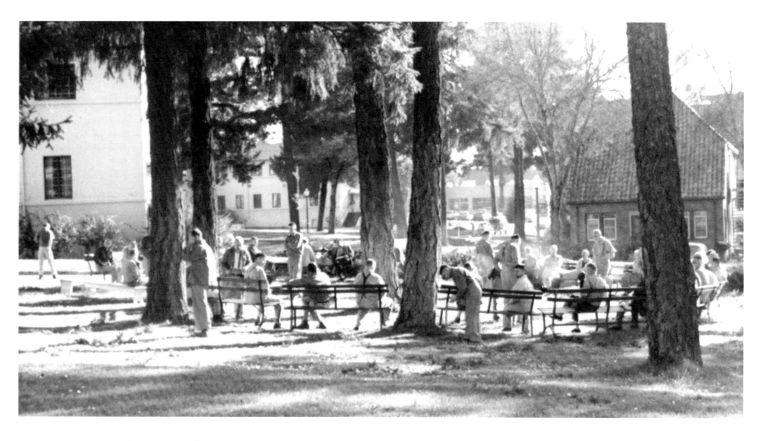

One of the state hospital's most profound effects on health care in Ukiah, in addition to the care it provided, was serving as a magnet for well-trained physician specialists who would otherwise never have come to the area. Ukiah was transitioning from the old model of care—a general practitioner and a nurse—to its first specialists, who needed time to build a practice. Employment at the state hospital provided the critical time they needed to do so.

The facility also served as a home for youth with no family and nowhere else to go. Ukiah resident Barbara Rones remembered receiving permission from the director of the youth program, Dr. Richard "Dick" Drury, to spend some time with the teens away from the premises. "These kids just needed someone to love them and pay attention, someone to nurture them and take them away for the afternoon," Rones said. She would pick them up once a week and take them out for ice cream or to her home to bake cookies so they could have a respite from their institutional surroundings.

In the 1960s, in response to a trend toward deinstitutionalization and in an effort to cut spending, California began to curtail state hospitals' offerings and closed many state psychiatric hospitals. The Lanterman-Petris-Short Act, signed into law by then-governor Ronald Reagan in 1967, was at the time considered a protection for those with mental illness by ending "inappropriate, indefinite, and involuntary commitment" and "safeguard[ing] individual rights." The bi-partisan act was passed by a wide margin and heralded by psychiatric advisors and reformers alike.[5]

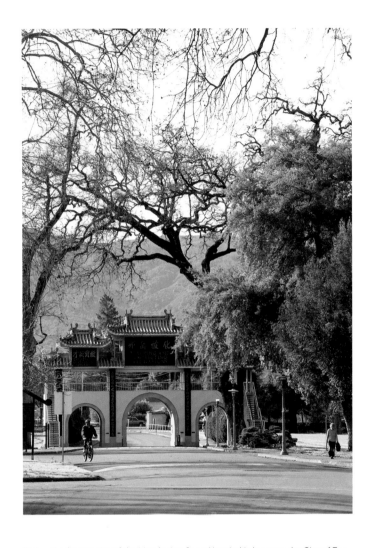

Today, the former site of the Mendocino State Hospital is home to the City of Ten Thousand Buddhas, a place of worship and education.

However, these professionals overestimated the effectiveness of new drugs and the ability of community clinics to care for mentally ill patients, so with the closure of the Mendocino State Hospital in 1972, more than a thousand patients in Mendocino County were left without adequate treatment. In addition to taking on the added burden of care, the county also lost $8 million in net dividends that had come from the facility's nine hundred fifty employees and their families.[6]

According to Ron Parker, a former hospital psychiatric technician and later a Mendocino County sheriff's deputy, the process of relocating and releasing patients took several years. Many long-term patients were transferred to facilities in Napa, Sonoma, Stockton, and Camarillo depending on their diagnoses and conditions. Others were reassigned to facilities in the community, which had been promised reimbursement monies for the patients' care; however, when the money was not forthcoming, the patients were released into the community. Parker became a deputy around this time and said he saw many former Mendocino State Hospital patients on the streets. He was the go-to guy when the Mendocino County Sheriff's Department was called to manage a situation involving a mentally ill person. Today local law enforcement personnel receive training on how to de-escalate potentially violent situations with mentally ill people who may not understand the consequences of their actions.

LANGLAND HOSPITAL

At the turn of the twentieth century, many communities had private hospitals in addition to government-sponsored hospitals; they were either for-profit hospitals or community-supported non-profit hospitals, some with religious affiliations. In Ukiah, the privately-owned Langland Hospital opened in 1913 on the corner of Spring and Stephenson Streets. Langland would not qualify as a hospital by modern standards, being nothing more than a renovated part of a nurse's home; however, it offered excellent care for its time.

When Cora Langland's husband passed away in 1911, she needed to support herself and her children. She decided to dedicate herself exclusively to hospital work; she was already a nurse, and in 1912 she spent a year in San Francisco obtaining additional training to prepare for life as a hospital nurse and administrator. When she returned to Ukiah, she opened Langland Hospital and offered the use of its "modern" operating room to local doctors, charging thirty dollars per week for confinement cases (hospitalization). The hospital steadily expanded, adding a ward in 1915 and a bungalow in 1920. According to Aurelius O. Carpenter and Percy H. Millberry in the *Histories of Lake and Mendocino Counties*, Mrs. Cora Langland was the "leader of an enterprise that from both philanthropic and financial standpoints is of importance to the city.... Through her practical ability as a nurse, combined with business efficiency of a high order, she is admirably qualified to establish and develop a hospital that will form a permanent asset in the public institutions of city and county." Little did they know how prescient their comments were, as Langland Hospital became the foundation for Ukiah General Hospital.

By 1921, Langland had married Dr. G. K. Osborn and ceded management of the hospital to Theresa Kramer Ray and her husband Sam Ray, who managed the hospital for two years. In 1922, the couple remodeled the facility, but Theresa Ray knew the hospital would not be able to keep up with the community's medical needs in the years to come, so she began raising funds to build a bigger, more modern hospital in Ukiah.

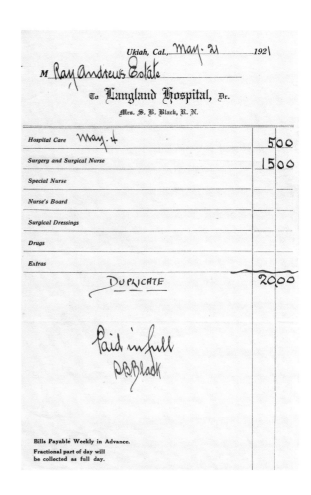

Nurse and administrator Cora Langland offered the use of her hospital's "modern" operating room to local doctors. This receipt from May 4, 1921, indicates a $20.00 charge for hospital care, surgery, and a surgical nurse. In 2016, that would be equal to $267.00.

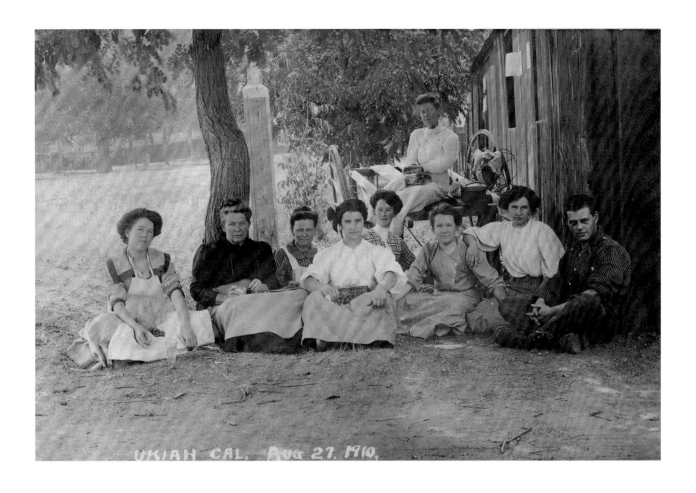

UKIAH CAL. Aug 27. 1910.

Above: Ukiah Steam Laundry, 1910. This photograph is an excellent depiction of the era during which both Lathrop Hospital and Langland Hospital provided care.

Right: Hop pickers at camp in Hopland, fifteen miles south of Ukiah, 1910.

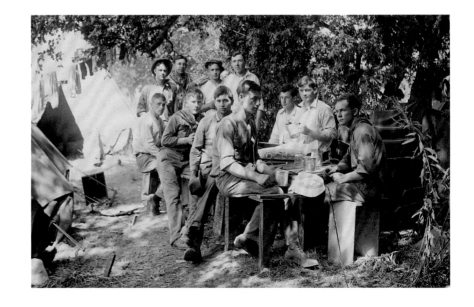

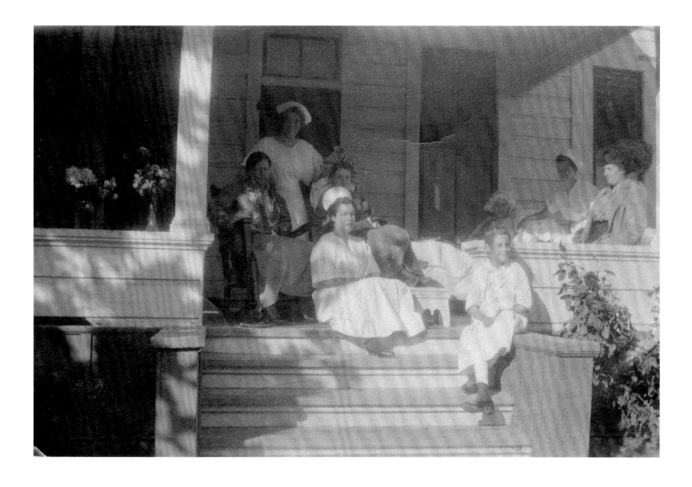

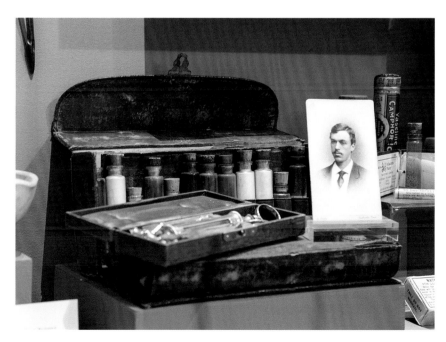

Above: Nurses from Langland Hospital took patients out on the porch for some fresh air and sunshine. At the corner of Spring and Stephenson Streets, the hospital opened with three beds in 1913.

Left: Dr. John Hudson's case of homeopathic medicines along with an 1880 photograph of the young physician from Nashville, Tennessee, on display in Ukiah's Grace Hudson Museum. Hudson arrived in Ukiah in 1889, working as a doctor for the San Francisco and North Pacific Railroad. He later left medicine to study Pomo peoples.

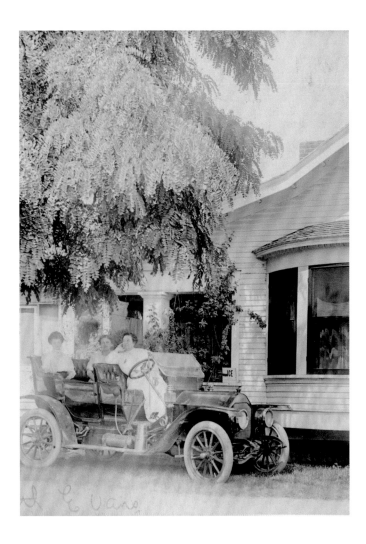

In 1902, Dr. Ida May Lathrop opened a hospital in her home. It was located just a few blocks away from where Langland Hospital would open ten years later. In the picture above, she sits in the driver's seat, parked in front of her hospital.

In 1928, the Langland Hospital building was sold and converted into apartments. By this time, Theresa Ray had poured her heart into raising money to build Ukiah General Hospital. The twenty-one-bed facility opened at 564 South Dora Street in August 1927.

Ukiah General Hospital

During the 1930s and '40s, Ukiah General Hospital, or "the General" as it was referred to, was the only private hospital in Ukiah, and it served the community well by standards of the day. This was due in no small part to Theresa Ray, its founder.

In recounting his early days in medicine in the 1940s, Dr. Glenn Miller described Ukiah General Hospital as a renovated house with twenty beds and one all-purpose room for surgeries, deliveries, and emergencies with walls so thin that the slightest groan from a woman in labor could be heard by family members down the hall. Even though the hospital had never been a residence, hospital floor plans in the late 1920s felt more like homes than hospitals by today's standards.

In 1946, nurses Myrtle Heise and Blanche Maher went in together to purchase General Hospital, and by 1955 they had added equipment, created a dietary department, and doubled the hospital's capacity from twenty to forty beds.

In 1959, after Maher's retirement, Heise bought out her partner's financial interest and became the sole owner, and the rule of "Iron Pants" began, according to family physician Dr. Robert Werra. "It was her way or the highway," he said. While she could be a little hard to get along with, her dedication to patients was unquestioned. "Her life was wrapped around the hospital patient," explained her son, Larry Heise. "In any big discussion, she wanted to know: how did the patient benefit from this?" Doctors said Heise was a taskmaster and careful with money, but they respected the "tough old bird," as obstetrician Dr. Vincent Valente called her.

Theresa Kramer Ray

PERSISTENCE PAYS

In the modern history of health care in Ukiah, few stand out as brightly as Theresa Kramer Ray, a nurse who convinced the town's citizens she could build a modern hospital—all they had to do was pay for it.

Born in Bremen, Germany, in 1896, Kramer came to America at age twelve to live with her aunt and uncle in New York, where she worked as a waitress in their restaurant, Grawbowsky's. Starting with the English phrases "come in" and "sit down," Kramer was able to speak English fluently within a year.

Her brothers served on merchant ships and visited often. When she shared her dream of going to California, her brother agreed to help her as long as Kramer agreed to live with a family of his choosing. This paved the way for her to move to San Francisco in 1914 and live with the Oliver Johanson family.

The Johansons treated Kramer as though she were their own daughter, appreciating her help in their dry goods store and in their home. When she developed a "felon" (infection) on her finger, Kramer was fascinated with the way the nurse dressed her wound. Afterward, she shared with Mrs. Johanson that she would like to become a nurse, so Mrs. Johanson made arrangements for Kramer to meet Dr. Manning, who then scheduled an interview for Kramer with the Fairmont Hospital's head nurse.

Kramer was taken on as a probationary nurse, scrubbing bedpans and other hospital equipment. Because of her work ethic and skill, she was eventually given additional responsibilities. She finished the three-year course of study to become a nurse, then continued her studies to become a surgical nurse.

It was then that her friend, Hilma Hansen, who had been managing Langland Hospital, asked Kramer to come to Ukiah to help her, but Kramer was not terribly interested. She agreed to visit Hansen in Ukiah to see this Langland Hospital, but it was not

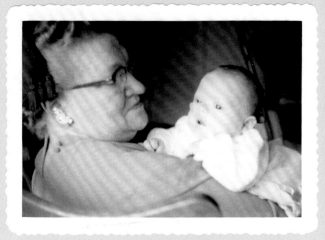

Theresa Ray in 1957, holding baby Steve, son of long-time friend Myrdell Watt. Ray was the driving force behind the building of Ukiah General Hospital years before.

until she saw the poor condition of the facility that she agreed to stay to help improve it. When Kramer gave notice at Fairmont Hospital, the administrator rejected her resignation and instead offered Kramer a year's leave of absence, confident she would return.

At Langland, Kramer modernized the operating room and assisted with surgeries and baby deliveries while Hansen managed the rest of the hospital. They paid seventy-five dollars a month in rent for the building, and that did not include provisions. Kramer took private nursing jobs to help pay for expenses and neither woman drew a salary, but still the hospital was not financially viable. After a year, Kramer returned to Fairmont Hospital, unaware that love was destined to make Ukiah her home.

The taxi driver who met Kramer at the train depot when she first arrived in Ukiah was Sam Ray, and he was smitten once he laid eyes on her. While she worked at Langland, Ray waited in front of the hospital for hours simply so he could visit with her for a few minutes each day. Just months after Kramer returned to San Francisco, she found Ray waiting for her as she left work; he had taken a job with a ship-building company in San Francisco, and he courted her each day when her workday was done.

In 1919 they were married, and their son, Sam Jr., was born a year later. They returned to Ukiah, and when little Sam was two years old, Kramer (now Ray) returned to Langland. Sam would play in the yard, where his mother could keep an eye on him while she attended to her nursing duties.

Within a short time, her concerns about Langland's inadequate facilities drove her to meet with Charles Mannon, president of the board at the Savings Bank of Mendocino County. She told him she wanted a loan to build a hospital, to which he replied, "What makes you think you can build a hospital?" After their conversation, the banker told her if she could raise $10,000 in subscriptions, he would match it.

In an interview printed in the *Ukiah Daily Journal* on February 15, 1972, Ray said, "I went to everyone in the community. I told them we were only borrowing the money and they would get it back. One sweet little Italian lady gave me $600.00. She said, 'I know I won't get it back, but we need a hospital.' I assured her she would get it back. She refused to believe me, but she wanted me to have the money anyway." As fate would have it, this woman's name was the first one drawn when it came time for subscribers to be repaid.

The new hospital opened in August 1927, and because of a terrible head-on train crash that killed both engineers, the facility was filled to capacity the day it opened; twenty-five patients were taken to the twenty-one-bed hospital.

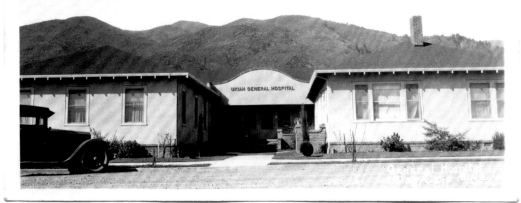

Ukiah General Hospital opened in 1927 on 564 South Dora Street. It had 15 hospital beds, plus living quarters for the owner.

In 1960, the hospital expanded to include a radiology department, a medical records department, and a conference room. In 1965, another renovation added a new patient wing, bringing the total capacity to forty-five beds. In 1970, Larry Heise followed in his mother's footsteps, becoming administrator of the General after having served as business manager and assistant administrator since 1960. According to Dr. Valente, Heise was a businessman, not a clinician, but, "Mr. Heise always supported us, not just with money, but with his attitude. He wanted the General to be the best hospital around."

The three local hospitals–Community, Hillside and General–continued to vie for patients during Mr. Heise's tenure, but now it became a fierce competition to prove which hospital had the most technically advanced equipment. The cost of this competition, combined with changes in reimbursement, reduced profits and led Heise and other small hospitals in the region to create a publicly held company, Ross Medical Group, in 1971; they hoped to gain efficiencies through economies of scale.

A year later, Hospital Corporation of America (HCA) purchased Ukiah General, and within a few years, HCA had financed the construction of the most expensive hospital in the country at the time–the high cost of the hospital was a result of being the first to comply with the new Alfred E. Alquist Hospital Seismic Safety Act. In explaining the seismic regulations, Heise said, "I am not exaggerating: The toaster that sat on the counter in the cafeteria had to be bolted down. The toilet paper holders in all the restrooms had to be certified by the manufacturer as being seismic safe. There were just innumerable requirements, but we got them all done, and we and Palm Drive were the first seismic-safe hospitals in the state." The new facility was located at 1120 South Dora Street, and it opened July 2, 1976.

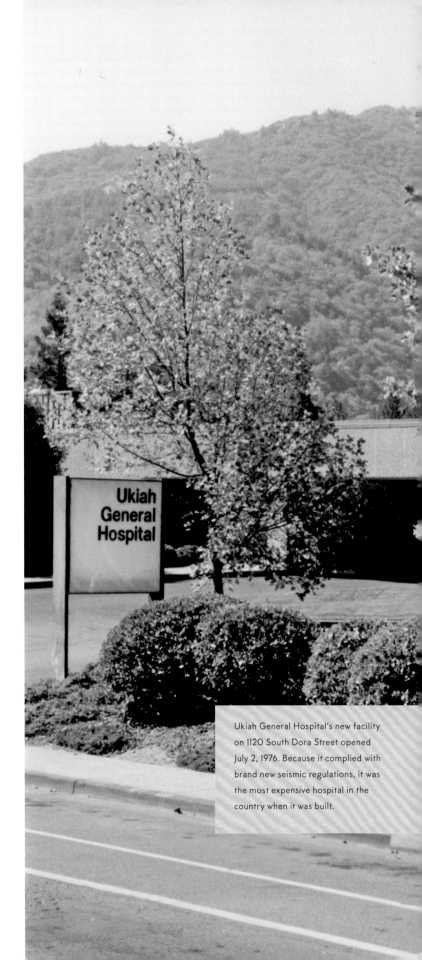

Ukiah General Hospital's new facility on 1120 South Dora Street opened July 2, 1976. Because it complied with brand new seismic regulations, it was the most expensive hospital in the country when it was built.

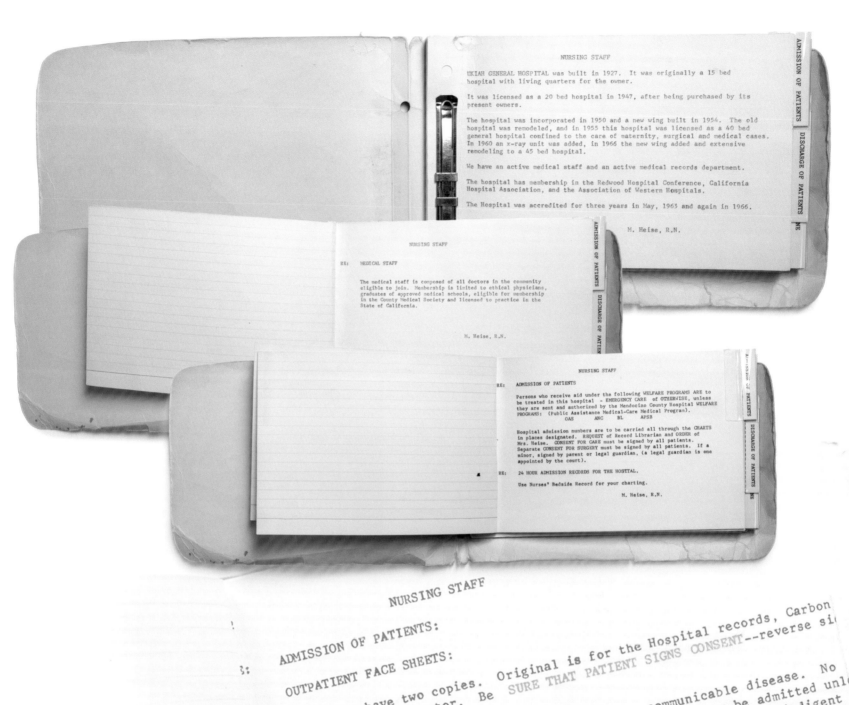

NURSING STAFF

UKIAH GENERAL HOSPITAL was built in 1927. It was originally a 15 bed hospital with living quarters for the owner.

It was licensed as a 20 bed hospital in 1947, after being purchased by its present owners.

The hospital was incorporated in 1950 and a new wing built in 1954. The old hospital was remodeled, and in 1955 this hospital was licensed as a 40 bed general hospital confined to the care of maternity, surgical and medical cases. In 1960 an x-ray unit was added, in 1966 the new wing added and extensive remodeling to a 45 bed hospital.

We have an active medical staff and an active medical records department.

The hospital has membership in the Redwood Hospital Conference, California Hospital Association, and the Association of Western Hospitals.

The Hospital was accredited for three years in May, 1963 and again in 1966.

M. Heise, R.N.

NURSING STAFF

RE: MEDICAL STAFF

The medical staff is composed of all doctors in the community eligible to join. Membership is limited to ethical physicians, graduates of approved medical schools, eligible for membership in the County Medical Society and licensed to practice in the State of California.

M. Heise, R.N.

NURSING STAFF

RE: ADMISSION OF PATIENTS

Persons who receive aid under the following WELFARE PROGRAMS ARE to be treated in this hospital - EMERGENCY CARE of OTHERWISE, unless they are sent and authorized by the Mendocino County Hospital WELFARE PROGRAMS: (Public Assistance Medical-Care Medical Program).
          OAS   ANC   BL   APSB

Hospital admission numbers are to be carried all through the CHARTS in places designated. REQUEST of Record Librarian and ORDER of Mrs. Heise. CONSENT FOR CARE must be signed by all patients. Separate CONSENT FOR SURGERY must be signed by all patients. If a minor, signed by parent or legal guardian, (a legal guardian is one appointed by the court).

RE: 24 HOUR ADMISSION RECORDS FOR THE HOSPITAL.

Use Nurses' Bedside Record for your charting.

M. Heise, R.N.

NURSING STAFF

ADMISSION OF PATIENTS:

OUTPATIENT FACE SHEETS:

... sure that you have two copies. Original is for the Hospital records, Carbon ... copy is for the doctor. Be SURE THAT PATIENT SIGNS CONSENT--reverse si... of original.

No patient shall be admitted suffering from a communicable disease. No ... drug addicts or alcoholics are admitted. No patient may be admitted unl... under the care of a doctor. All emergencies are accepted. If indigent ... will be transferred to the County Hospital when able to be transferred or ... on order from the doctor.

The business office shall take charge of all admissions. When the offic... is closed the registered nurse on duty shall have charge of the admissi... of all patients. All information data must be complete. Look at the ... Rules and Regulations sheets posted on your Bulletin Boards.

M. Heise, R.N.

Above: The booklet was titled, "Nursing Staff Rules and Regulations" and it outlined Ukiah General Hospital's guidelines.

Opposite: Myrtle Heise passes on the shovel to son Larry Heise after breaking ground on Ukiah General Hospital's new site at 1120 South Dora Street.

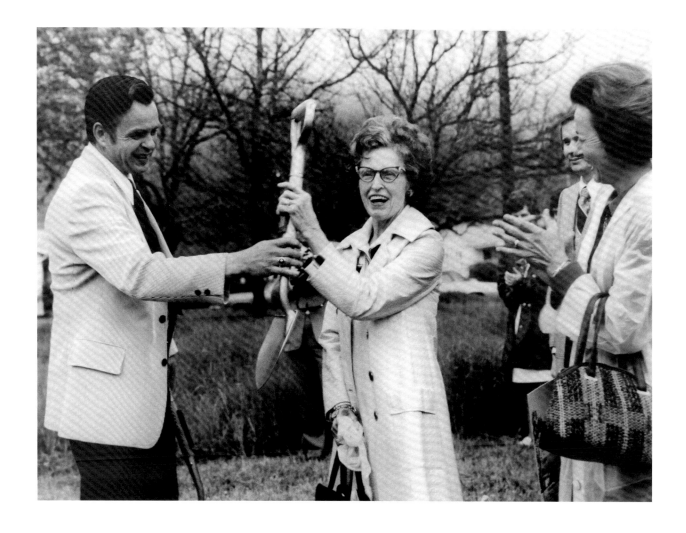

A year later [1972], Hospital Corporation of America (HCA) purchased Ukiah General, and within a few years, HCA had financed the construction of the most expensive hospital in the country at the time—the high cost of the hospital was a result of being the first to comply with the new Alfred E. Alquist Hospital Seismic Safety Act.

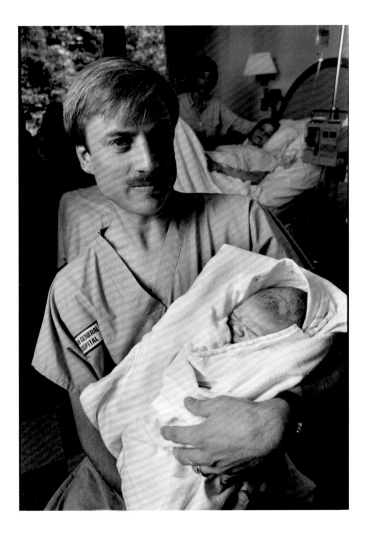

The caption on the back of this photograph from 1989 explains why Dr. Jerrel Emery is holding the last public-assistance delivery he would perform locally. It stated, "Local ob-gyn group stopped taking Medi-Cal patients...Two obstetricians moved to more populated areas for bigger salaries and less hectic workloads. Welfare mothers now must drive to a large city in another county for care."

Having access to modern medical technology was great for many in Ukiah's medical community, but having two private hospitals and a public hospital seemed like a duplication of resources; medical professionals argued that Ukiah would be better served by one large hospital to care for everyone. It would be years, however, before only one hospital remained open.

Many of the doctors who practiced at Ukiah General look back on their work there with fondness. Dr. Valente recalled with pride the fact that only 10 percent of Ukiah General's at-risk deliveries were rerouted to Santa Rosa or San Francisco, and oncologist and pathologist Dr. Herschel Gordon enjoyed sharing his role in founding Ukiah General's local blood bank.

Dr. Gordon said that in the early 1980s he asked hospital administrator Kelly Morgan if he could start a blood bank, and Morgan said, "Hey, you want to do a blood bank? Great. It's a good idea. Good publicity. Good for our hospital. Good for our community." Competitors from Sonoma County tried to undermine the new venture's credibility, but Dr. Gordon's good reputation and strong relationships with out-of-the-area blood banks helped end the Sonoma County competitors' monopoly in Mendocino County.

As the 1980s wore on, hospitals had to pay more attention to the bottom line and balance the needs and desires of patients, doctors, allied health professionals, and employees. HCA was a for-profit national powerhouse in the hospital business, and it expanded quickly during the 1970s. However, by the 1980s, it began to contract, selling assets in the west and consolidating its holdings in the eastern part of the country. When profits at Ukiah General dwindled, HCA decided to sell, which they eventually did in 1988.

At that time, General Hospital's rival was Hillside Community Hospital, which was owned by Adventist Health System/West. Adventist Health and HCA each owned hospitals in both Ukiah and a town in Tennessee. General Hospital's chief of staff at the time, Dr. Larry Falk, understood there to be an agreement between the two organizations whereby Adventist Health would take ownership of the Ukiah General property and HCA would take ownership of Adventist Health's hospital in Tennessee.

According to obstetrical nurse Nyota Wiles, Ukiah General employees thought they would be involved in decisions about the sale of their hospital because they believed HCA made corporate decisions with employee input. This was not the case with regard to the General, however. When HCA sold Ukiah General's assets to Adventist Health, many employees who worked for the General struggled with the decision because they did not want to work for their competitor, so much so that after August 8, 1988, when Adventist Health acquired the assets of Ukiah General Hospital, doctors from the General banded together to fight the sale. They brought a lawsuit against Adventist Health under the Clayton Antitrust Act and traveled to San Francisco to participate in Federal Trade Commission hearings.

Eventually the FTC ruled in favor of Adventist Health. The blending of the two hospitals was one of the biggest events in Ukiah's health care history. While there were many benefits to having only one hospital—less duplication, streamlined processes, improved communication—it took years for hard feelings to subside. Doctors who had just sued Adventist Health now needed to care for patients there. Employees loyal to Adventist Health-run Hillside had trouble understanding why those from the General struggled with the culture of their new employer. It took a long time for "us" and "them" to become "we."

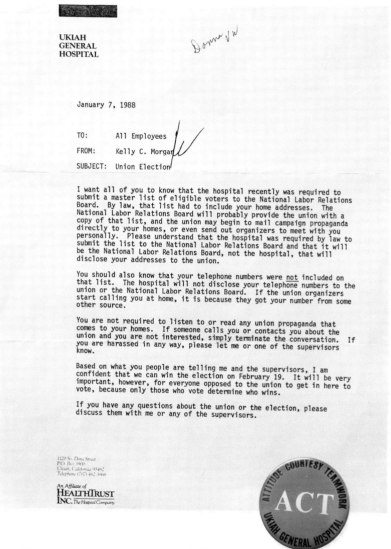

Top: 1988 was a tumultuous year for health care in Ukiah.

Bottom: A pin worn by Ukiah General Hospital employees.

A Brief History of Adventist Health

Because some of Hillside Community Hospital's influential founders and staff were members of the Seventh-day Adventist Church, the hospital came to follow many of the church's teachings as they related to health care.

Since the mid-1800s, the Seventh-day Adventist Church has advocated for a healthy lifestyle involving good nutrition (extolling the virtues of a vegetarian diet), exercise, and hygiene as a means of preventing illness. In fact, when women's fashion dictated long skirts, the Adventists recommended what was considered by some to be a scandalous idea—lifting hemlines above the ankles to pull skirts out of the horse manure and other muck. Adventists such as surgeon and

nutritionist Dr. John Harvey Kellogg also bucked tradition in favor of health, replacing the common ham and eggs breakfast of the times with his creation of Corn Flakes in 1878.

Adventists set up sanitariums from Michigan to California, which, a century later, led to the creation of Adventist Health Services (AHS) in 1972. In 1980, AHS restructured and became Adventist Health System/West incorporating several western states, and eventually simply "Adventist Health." Hillside Community Hospital eventually became Ukiah Adventist Hospital (UAH) to better represent its affiliation with Adventist Health.

Surgical procedures changed dramatically from the inception of Adventist Health to the current day.

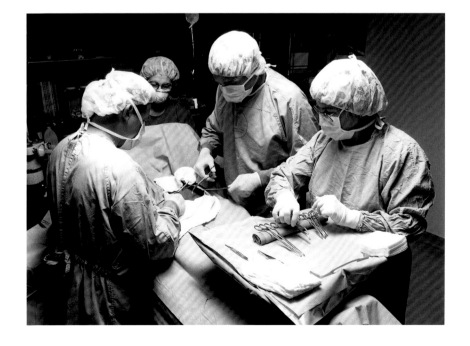

HILLSIDE COMMUNITY HOSPITAL

While some physicians loved working at Ukiah General Hospital in the 1950s, other physicians wanted their own hospital. The man primarily responsible for building Hillside Community Hospital on Laws Avenue in Ukiah was Dr. Robert Barr, and the first board of directors, which included many investors, was comprised of chairman Dr. Neal Woods, Dr. Carl Aagaard, Dr. Barr, Dr. James Massengill, and Dr. Les Provencher. Other early investors included Dr. Cloice Biggins, Dr. Glenn Miller, and Dr. Nicholas Zbitnoff.

In January 1956, nurse Shirley Ann Munroe, who had been working for Dr. Barr, began preparing for the opening of the new hospital. She and fellow nurse Florence Foster from Lakeside Hospital in neighboring Lakeport, California, helped select and order hospital furnishings and equipment. The two women traveled to San Francisco to buy everything from "desks and wastebaskets to bedstands and bedpans," according to Munroe. By September, hospital hallways were lined with boxes that took a month to unpack and organize.

Hillside Community Hospital opened its doors on October 14, 1956, and the first patient arrived two days later, causing "utter pandemonium," according to Munroe. Many employees had never worked in a hospital before, and policies and procedures were still under development. Simple questions arose, such as did patient identification bracelets belong on the left wrist or the right? What was the proper order for pages in a patient's medical chart?

When it opened, the hospital had forty-four patient beds, two operating rooms, X-ray and laboratory services, a therapy unit, and a four-bed pediatric ward. Modern conveniences included patient-operated pillow radio speakers, a patient-to-desk speaker system, and telephones in the

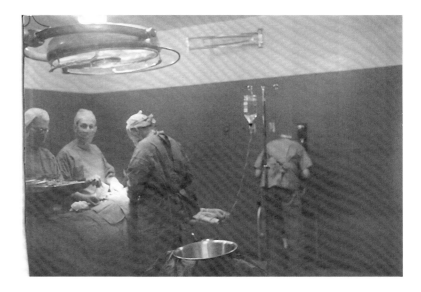

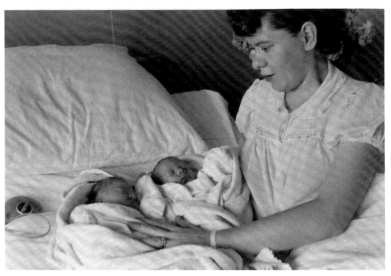

Top: This is the first surgery performed at Hillside Community Hospital in 1956. Note the glass IV bottle; now plastic bags are used to hold IV fluids.

Bottom: These were the first twins born at Hillside Community Hospital: Cheryl and Carol Lewis born December 6, 1956.

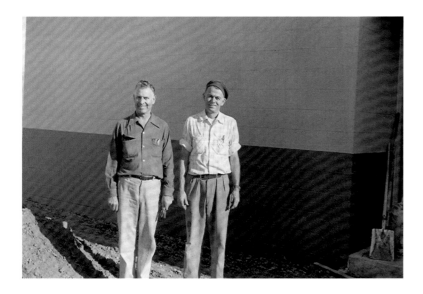

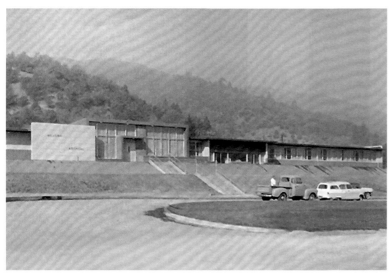

Top: Slater, Penner & Wilson was the contracting company that built Hillside Community Hospital in 1956. (Left: Mr. Slater, Right: Woody Wilson). When Dr. Robert Barr ran out of money half way through construction, other doctors in town joined together to fund the hospital's completion. The contractors building the hospital also hit hard times. Mike Wilson, son of contractor Woody Wilson, reminisced about the generosity of the Frassinello family who owned Johnnie's Market on Observatory and State Streets. The Frassinellos allowed his father "to run up a bill for a couple years" so he could feed his family.

Bottom: This is the earliest known photograph of the newly-built Hillside Community Hospital, taken shortly after it opened in 1956.

Opposite: Hillside Community Hospital and Ukiah General Hospital competed for patients and employees, promoting their excellence as hospitals and places to work.

twelve semi-private patient rooms. Each of these rooms could be converted into two private rooms.

Upon the hospital's opening, Munroe slept in the nurses' lounge for two weeks to be sure someone knowledgeable was available to answer questions day and night, and Dr. Provencher was the hospital administrator for the first nine months. After that, Munroe took over as administrator and secretary to the board of directors. Jeanne Mooney was the hospital's head nurse, and the medical staff consisted of twenty-three doctors from Ukiah, Willits, and Lakeport, with Dr. Neely Bradford of Boonville serving as chief of staff.[7]

Like Myrtle Heise, Munroe was a skilled administrator who was respected but whose commanding and autocratic style was not always appreciated. Dorothy Bowen, RN, Hillside's operating room nurse supervisor in the 1950s and '60s, said, "Shirley Ann could be a fly in the ointment. She tended to stir up feelings of animosity between the hospitals, but I respected her role as administrator."

From the moment Hillside Hospital opened, it was in a "ferocious shootout" with Ukiah General Hospital, according to family practitioner Dr. Peter Keegan, who began his career in Ukiah at Mendocino Community Hospital. Physicians, especially surgeons, typically aligned themselves with one hospital or the other, and their loyalty was often rewarded with preferred access to that hospital's operating room. Surgical procedures commanded excellent reimbursement, so the hospitals competed for surgeons' loyalty for the next thirty years. Community members also typically aligned with one hospital or the other, so many physicians simply asked their patients where they would prefer to receive care, as nearly all the physicians had privileges at both facilities. While the competition was fierce at times, the two hospitals

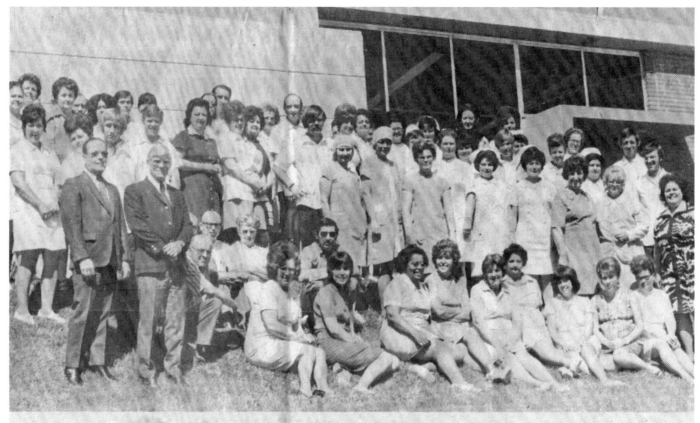

Day shift employees at Hillside Community Hospital of Ukiah.
Approximately 60c of every dollar in the hospital budget is used to pay employee wages and salaries. The average hotel employs one person for every six guests. To provide a full range of services around the clock for six patients, the average hospital must employ 13.3 personnel.

From the moment Hillside Hospital opened, it was in a "ferocious shootout" with Ukiah General Hospital.... Physicians, especially surgeons, typically aligned themselves with one hospital or the other, and their loyalty was rewarded with preferred access to that hospital's operating room.

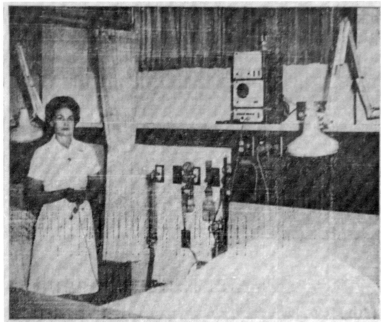

LIFE-SAVING UNIT—More than 300 persons Sunday got a close look at Hillside Community Hospital's unique self-contained Intensive Care-Coronary Care four-bed addition, which will provide 24-hour intensive care for critically ill patients. Supervisor Carolyn Brown is shown by one of the four recessed bedside panels which contain outlets for emergency thoracic, abdominal and tracheal suction, compressed air, oxygen and helium used in care of critically ill patients. Each bed is electrically raised; each patient's respiratory and vital functions, including heart beat, can be controled by a pacemaker and a monitor-screen above the bed. Two especially trained nurses will be on duty at all times and can care for four patients at once, with help of electronic controls.

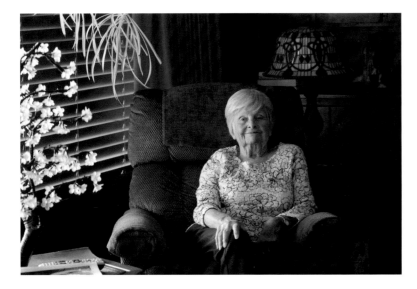

collaborated for the good of their patients. Bowen recalled the two hospitals regularly sharing instruments. "There was no animosity between departments. My loyalty was to Hillside, but the ORs were friendly. We loaned instruments all the time," she said.

As Hillside expanded, the technology it employed grew increasingly advanced. Ads often highlighted the latest equipment acquisition as a reason to choose one hospital over another. An ad in the 1959 *Ukiah News* boasted Hillside as having thirteen active doctors and sixteen courtesy doctors, 2,285 patients, and 289 babies since opening, and was "now offering the most complete X-ray unit available, the famous Picker X-ray unit with fluoroscopic attachment."

Hillside Hospital received accreditation from the Joint Commission on the Accreditation of Healthcare Organizations in 1961. In 1966, it became a non-profit hospital and added a licensed vocational nursing program. The hospital continued to expand, adding an intensive care unit with a separate nursing station in 1968, respiratory therapy in 1969, the community's first physical therapy department in 1970, a licensed pharmacy in 1972, a nuclear medicine department in 1974, and the community's first twenty-four-hour, physician-staffed emergency department in 1975.

By the mid-1970s, seismic and life safety regulations made building a new facility more attractive than retrofitting the existing facility,[8] but not everyone in the community was enthusiastic about a new hospital. With the recent building of a new General Hospital, community doctors and local politicians expressed concerns that another new facility would lead to higher prices and less efficient health care for patients. In their view, continued competition between Hillside and General would result in unnecessary duplication of services and equipment.[9] However, those in favor of building a new, modern facility prevailed, and construction moved forward with the help of Adventist Health Services (AHS), who purchased Hillside hospital in late 1978 at Munroe's request. Erwin Remboldt, then president of AHS said, "Hillside approached us so they could have the advantage of a multi-hospital system, which provides many savings to a hospital in purchasing, insurance, and management expertise."[10] In March 1980, patients were transferred from the old Hillside facility to the newly built and newly named Ukiah Adventist Hospital at East Perkins Street between North Orchard Street and Mason Street, on the aptly named Hospital Drive.

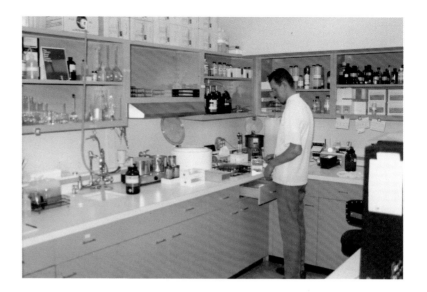

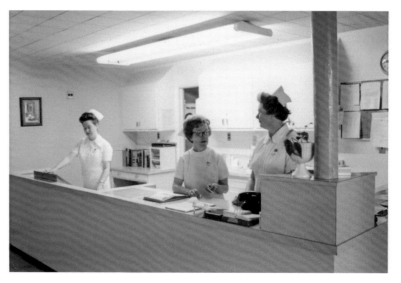

Top: Lab Director Orlando Knittle works in his lab at Hillside Community Hospital in 1971.

Bottom: This is the Hillside Community Hospital nurses' station circa 1971—no computers, only paper charts and telephones to record data and communicate. Left: Jennie Ward, LVN; Right: Lorrain Tollini, LVN; (nurse in the center was not identified).

Opposite Top: Carolyn Ford Brown, RN, attended nursing school as part of the US Cadet Program and then enjoyed a long nursing career in Ukiah.

Opposite Bottom: Carolyn Brown, RN, enjoys retirement in 2016.

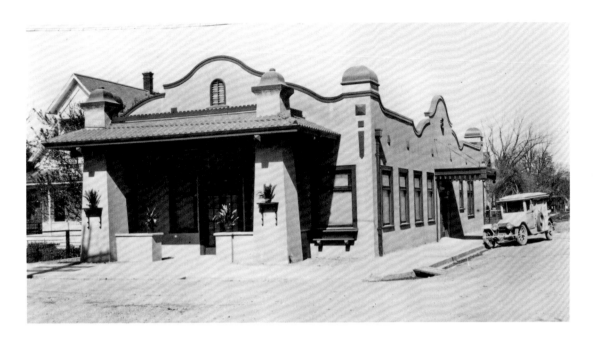

Top: Eversole Mortuary had a hearse that also served as an ambulance (note it parked to the right of the building). The mortuary was located at the northwest corner of School and Henry Streets in the 1920s, formerly the site of the Marks Opera House.

Middle: Air ambulances have saved many lives in Mendocino County's rough and rural terrain, often bringing patients to Ukiah Valley Medical Center.

Bottom: Ukiah Ambulance, later called Med-Star, is Ukiah's oldest local ambulance company, tracing its origins to 1937 when volunteer groups such as the Veterans of Foreign Wars, American Legion, 20-30 Club, and the Druids, came together to provide emergency medical transportation.

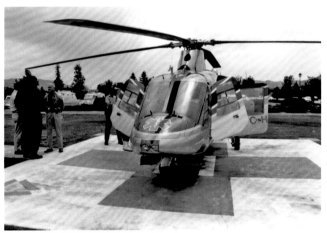

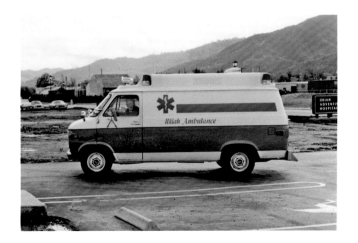

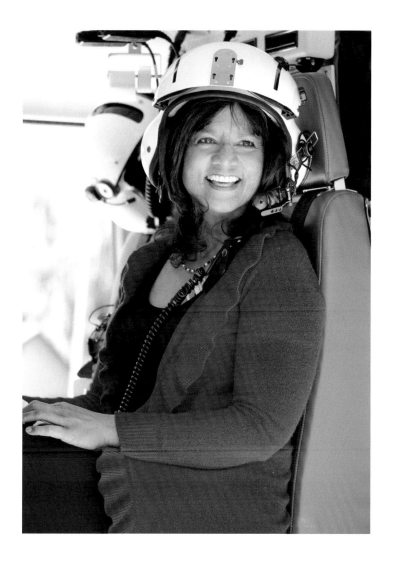

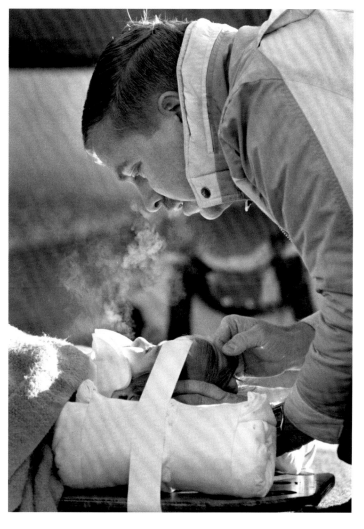

From the Eversole Mortuary hearse that doubled as an ambulance to the CALSTAR helicopter, emergency first responders often provide care that means the difference between life and death.

Left: Ukiah Valley Medical Center president Gwen Matthews enjoys a moment in the California Shock Trauma Air Rescue (CALSTAR) helicopter during a 2013 public event. CALSTAR has been serving Ukiah and the surrounding area since 1983.

Right: Ukiah Fire paramedic Norman "Chuck" Yates stabilizes a pediatric patient.

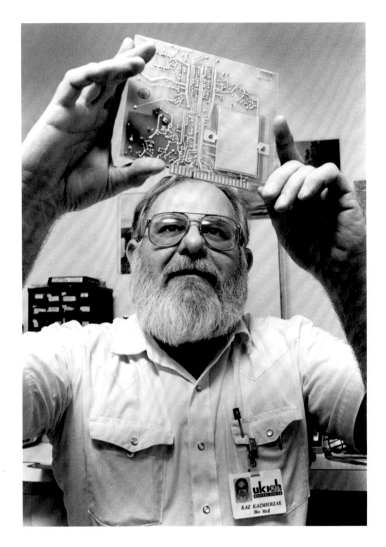

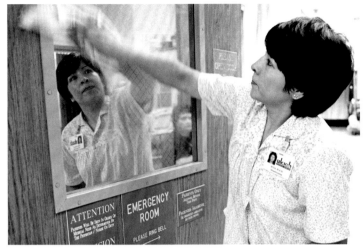

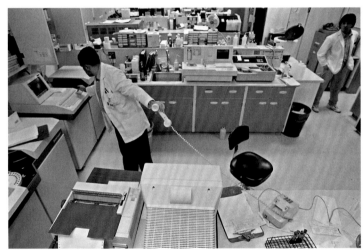

Left: Bio Tech expert Kaz Kazmierzak assures hospital equipment remains in good working order. He also played Santa at the hospital's annual employee Christmas party for years.

Top Right: Housekeeper Rosa Rojas cleans to keep the hospital safe and infection-free, a challenging task given the nature of hospital work.

Bottom Right: Lab Director Frank Walker tests the stretching capability of the phone cord as he checks on some information. Lab technician Chan Kajla looks on from the side.

Throughout the 1980s, three hospitals shared patients in Ukiah: Mendocino Community Hospital, owned by the county; Ukiah General Hospital, owned by HCA; and Ukiah Adventist Hospital, owned by AHS. By the 1990s, only Ukiah Adventist was still operating.

Ukiah Adventist Hospital

Throughout the 1980s, three hospitals shared patients in Ukiah: Mendocino Community Hospital, owned by the county; Ukiah General Hospital, owned by HCA; and Ukiah Adventist Hospital, owned by AHS. By the 1990s, only Ukiah Adventist was still operating.

In 1983, changes in federal reimbursement dramatically reduced hospital payments when Medicare and Medicaid moved from cost-based reimbursement to a prospective payment system based on diagnosis-related groups (DRGs). This new system limited what the government would pay for hospital care by standardizing treatment costs based on a patient's diagnosis. No longer could hospitals charge whatever it cost them to provide care and expect to be reimbursed for it. Instead, the DRG system paid hospitals a flat fee for a specific number of hospital days for each admitting diagnosis. Federal reimbursement for health care began to dictate, to some degree, how medicine would be practiced, because without federal money, hospitals could not afford to keep their doors open.

About this same time, and likely related to the need to control costs, hospital care was broken down into its component parts and became more task-oriented than patient-oriented. If a nurse's license allowed her to perform a task and it was less expensive for the nurse to do so rather than the doctor, the nurse or another licensed caregiver took care of it. Hospitals wanted everyone to work to the top of their licenses. The unintended result was that patients saw far more hospital caregivers but felt less connected to any of them. One person would manage bathing and the bedpan. Another would monitor vital signs. Another would deliver meals. Another would clean the

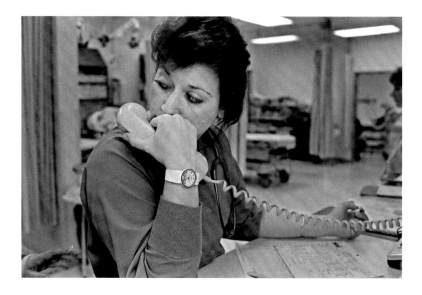

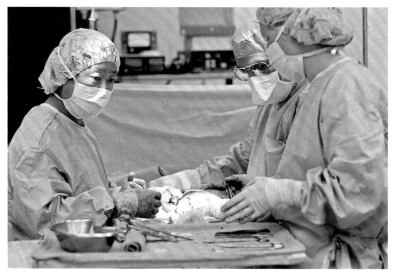

Top: Emergency room nurses like Edrina Kolling (pictured) were often faced with difficult decisions that had to be made relatively quickly if patients were to have the best chance of survival.

Bottom: A surgical team delivers a baby via cesarean section.

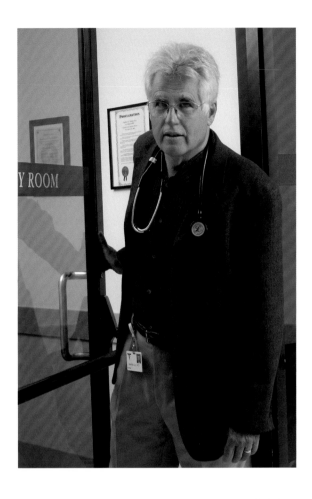

Years after Ukiah Adventist Hospital purchased the assets of Ukiah General Hospital, cardiologist Dr. Dale Morrison became the chief of staff and helped reduce animosity between the doctors from the two hospitals.

room. Another would provide transportation for lab or imaging tests. Another would oversee specialized issues regarding therapy or discharge. And then the doctor would check in. This could make finding the appropriate person to answer their questions difficult for patients and family members.

Everyone was watching the bottom line. Registered nurse Candy Gorbenko shared how financial concerns changed procedures in the operating room, explaining that in the early days, operating room nurses prepared for surgical cases by opening sterilized containers of instruments that the surgeon might want for the case. As the hospital became more cost conscious, this system was viewed as expensive and wasteful, so nurses changed their procedures by opening only the instruments and equipment they were certain would be used; the rest remained within arm's reach and could be opened if needed. See "The Law of Unintended Consequences" in the appendix for more information on how health care is affected by how it is funded.

Ukiah Valley Medical Center

When Ukiah Adventist Hospital (UAH) purchased the assets of Ukiah General Hospital on August 8, 1988, many people, including employees at both hospitals, believed the General had been in a stronger financial position and were shocked by the announcement. A year later, Ukiah Adventist Hospital was renamed Ukiah Valley Medical Center (UVMC).

While the facilities were repurposed and blended to meet the needs of the community, attitudes took longer to adjust. Tensions remained high, so much so that shortly after the hospitals came together, a doctor from General Hospital stood in the hospital waiting room, which was full of patients, and publicly insulted all UAH doctors, questioning the quality of their care as well as their integrity. Admitting Manager Betty Hook, who worked at UAH from 1967 to 1998, said she had to use considerable control not to respond in front of everyone. Instead she told hospital president ValGene Devitt what happened. After a conversation with Devitt, the doctor apologized.

During the 1990s, UVMC grew in size and scope as it cared for the whole community. By the mid-1990s, the hospital was one of the

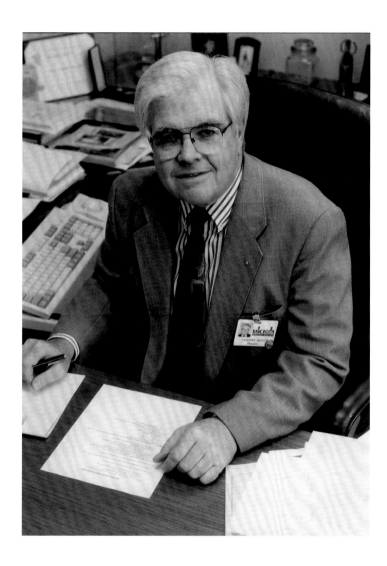

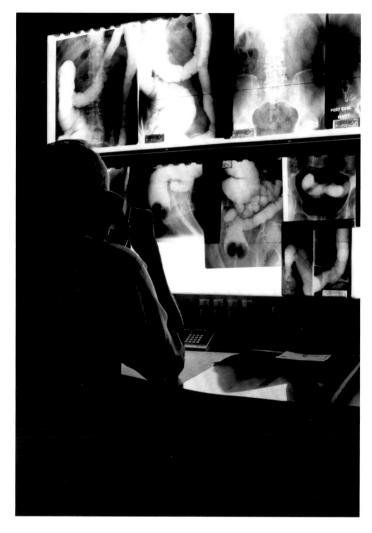

Ukiah Valley Medical Center president ValGene Devitt was at the helm when Ukiah General and Ukiah Adventist became one on August 8, 1988.

Above: Ukiah Valley Medical Center president ValGene Devitt oversaw the building of a new birthing center, repurposed the Dora Street site as a transitional care unit, and tried to help employees from two hospitals feel like one big hospital family.

Right: Radiologists like Dr. Gary Ballard spent many hours reviewing films on a view box in a dark room. Today, radiologists view digitized images on computer screens.

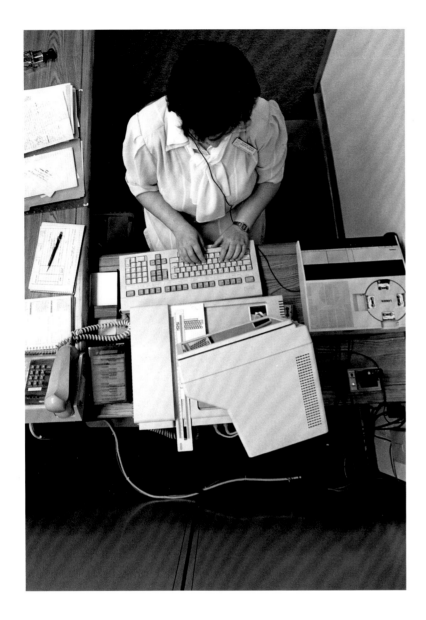

Transcriptionists listened to doctors' dictation and typed surgical reports, radiology reports, pathology reports, and more. The machine on the right side of the picture holds four mini-cassette tapes and the transcriptionist could slow down the doctors' dictation to capture every word.

biggest employers in Ukiah, with approximately 600 employees managing more than 70,000 patient visits per year. A contentious relationship between hospital administration and the medical staff, along with the nurses threatening to organize under the California Nurses Association, made it difficult for Devitt to accomplish many of his goals, but he worked toward them nonetheless. He oversaw the building of a new birthing center and repurposed the Dora Street property to make it a transitional care facility that provided patients with short-term rehabilitative care after their hospital stay.

The hospital also provided charity care and financial support to the community. In addition to making some hospital services available at little or no cost, UVMC sponsored free health classes, supported community events, encouraged employees to donate to the community through the United Way, and helped finance health-related endeavors, such as the county's community health status report.

As the twenty-first century dawned, Mark LaRose replaced ValGene Devitt as hospital president. LaRose came to Ukiah with a financial background, and his attempts to maximize profits caused hard feelings among many local physicians, in part because of contracts that provided benefits to some doctors and not others; also, many physicians felt their contributions were not appropriately valued as LaRose worked to reduce the cost of contracted services. The most contentious issues included paying for hospital Emergency Call (the system that assures doctors in certain medical specialties are available to the emergency department within twenty minutes), creating a federally designated rural health center with only one local medical group (allowing for higher reimbursement for Medi-Cal patients), and negotiating contracted services, such as emergency and radiology.

When Terry Burns arrived to take over as hospital president in 2007, however, wounds began to heal—both recent ones and those inflicted by the old General versus Hillside rivalry. Burns worked with the newly appointed chief of staff, cardiologist Dr. Dale Morrison, and together these two men helped bring years of anger and resentment to an end. Dr. Morrison invited doctors to share their concerns, and he put issues out in the open where they could be addressed. After learning which doctors did not support the hospital, Burns immediately invited them into his office and asked, "How can we work together? How can I help you be successful?" Dr. Larry Falk later recalled that, after being made to feel like a criminal by previous administrations for publicly disagreeing with hospital decisions, he was relieved and grateful for Burns' approach. "After he invited me into his office like that, I would do anything for him," Dr. Falk said. And so began the healing.

While individuals continued to disagree from time to time, collaboration among disparate parties became more frequent. Burns fostered this collaboration in the hospital and in the community. He formed a group of community leaders to tackle intractable and polarizing problems, and he named the group the Mustard Seed Coalition. Sheriff Tom Allman was a member. He said Burns came to the first meeting and told everyone, "The quality of life of these people who are in and out of our emergency room has to be improved, and if we don't improve it, nobody's going to improve it. It's up to us." The Mustard Seed discussions eventually led to the Chronic Users System of Care (CUSOC), a pilot project that demonstrated how treatment that included intensive case management could simultaneously be less expensive while producing better outcomes for patients. Patients who had suffered from addiction and mental illness, as well as chronic medical problems, were able to get their health under control. They stopped bouncing from the hospital to the jail to the Federally Qualified Health Center and back again, and they began living more productive lives.

After Burns left in 2011, registered nurse Gwen Matthews took over as UVMC's president and chief executive officer. The situation she walked into was enormously challenging, but she trusted that her experience and her integrity would see her through.

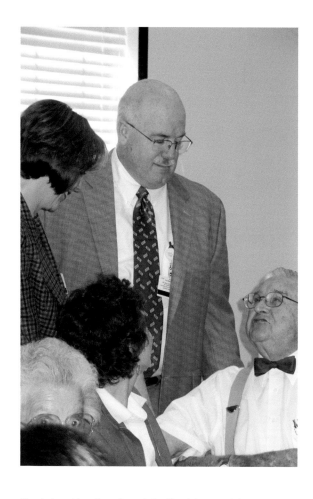

Hospital president Terry Burns helped heal the wounds between Ukiah General loyalists and Hillside Community Hospital loyalists. He wore his heart on his sleeve and encouraged open, honest communication. He is pictured here with Human Resources Director Cindy Wysong-Brown (standing on left) and hospital volunteer Dan Cornforth (seated on the right).

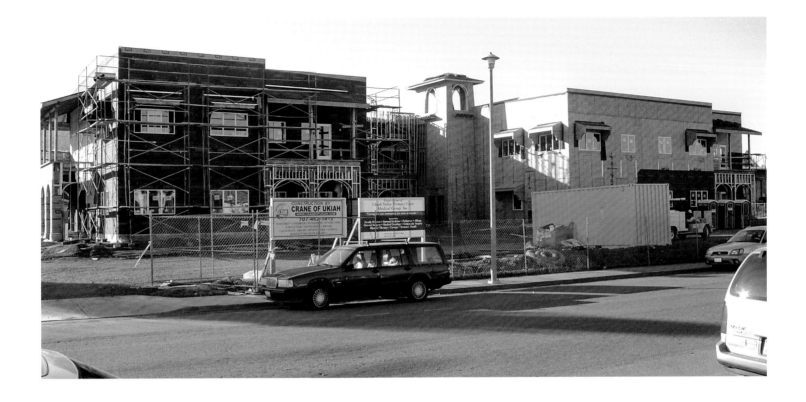

Above: The medical office building directly across the street from Ukiah Valley Medical Center was built to house the Rural Health Clinic. Adventist Health contracted with Ukiah Valley Primary Care to provide patient care.

Right: Modern operating rooms suspend lights and other equipment from the ceiling to allow for maximum flexibility of movement during surgeries.

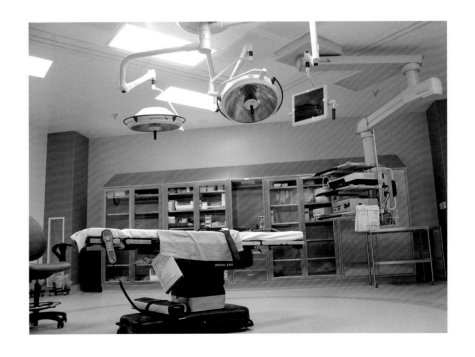

Gwen Matthews, RN, MSc, MBA

AN ADMINISTRATOR ON A MISSION

When Matthews arrived in Ukiah in 2011, not only had the hospital experienced financial losses in seven of the nine preceding months, but a few weeks before she arrived, an attorney told her about significant payments in arrears from the Outpatient Surgery Center—a joint venture in which the hospital participated with many local doctors—an issue that needed to be addressed immediately. Financial concerns mounted as Matthews received news that the Centers for Medicare and Medicaid Services (CMS) would be reducing annual payments to UVMC by $4 million, and additional federal payment reductions resulting from the Affordable Care Act (ACA) were predicted to make acute care unsustainable in six California counties—including Lake and Mendocino Counties, the two counties served by UVMC.

Matthews knew she would need all of her education and experience to improve UVMC's financial health. As a seasoned nurse executive, she understood hospital operations, and her MBA gave her a solid background in business and finance, but to get the hospital back on track, Matthews needed the trust and cooperation of her hospital team and the medical staff at a time when she had little to offer but formidable challenges and unpleasant news. The doctors who had invested in the surgery center felt their trust had recently been betrayed by hospital administrators and were in no mood to trust Matthews. From the monthly financial reports they had seen, it appeared the surgery center was breaking even when, in fact, it was $2.5 million in debt. The last UVMC CEO to make significant changes to improve the bottom line did not last long and was not well received, but Matthews believed that by coming from a place of transparency and integrity, with a firm commitment to the care of those UVMC served, a path could be found.

Within weeks of her arrival, Matthews began showing her hospital team and the medical staff what she was made of. After studying plans for a new emergency department and intensive

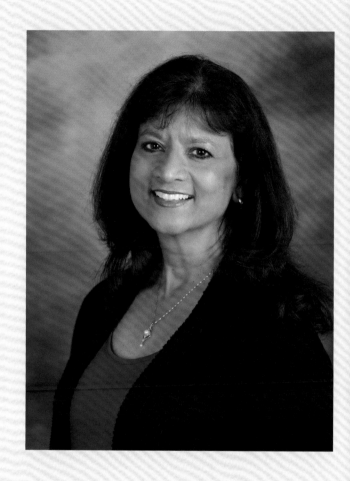

Hospital president Gwen Matthews overcame suspicion and distrust to become one of Ukiah Valley Medical Center's most respected leaders.

care unit, she found significant design flaws and she realized that construction would unnecessarily block all major hospital entrances for the entire construction period. Matthews could not allow plans to go forward without exploring additional options, but she understood the Adventist Health corporate office might not approve the capital funding required for a better complete plan.

Doctors who had been waiting for a new emergency department for years were furious. They worried that changes at this point would delay the project, and that Matthews' request for revisions might be a move to derail the project completely. Matthews told them that if she had not brought these issues to their attention, she would have been irresponsible. She explained that her choices and actions would always be based on what was best for the long-term service of the community, and if this meant they did not want her to lead the hospital, she would be happy to step down so someone else could do so. What she was unwilling to do this time—and every time—was to allow poor decisions to be made simply to avoid uncomfortable conversations or more hard work. How, in good conscience, could she not bring to light her concerns along with a plan to address them?

The doctors took a collective deep breath and decided to see if she would back up her rhetoric with action. She did. Once they understood the rationale for the new plans and recognized that they would have a better facility to serve the community for decades to come, they were supportive.

Matthews carried on what Burns had begun in terms of openness to those with dissenting ideas and a commitment to working together for the good of the whole Ukiah community. At a retirement party honoring his forty-two years of service in 2015, pathologist Dr. Herschel Gordon made a point of seeking out Matthews. He told her he had seen many administrators come and go but that none had stabilized hospital administration the way she had. He praised her consistency and told her how much he appreciated her approach. She responded, "Thank you. When I became president, I vowed to myself that any decisions we made would not be for the short term, but for the long run, so that long after I'm gone people might not know where the roots are, but I would have the satisfaction of knowing we had laid a solid foundation for whatever was needed to serve the community for the next forty or fifty years."

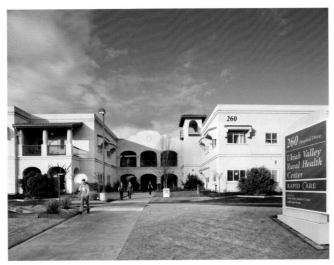

Gwen Matthews continued to promote health care in Ukiah through inpatient and outpatient care, as well as promoting local partnerships and street medicine.

One of the ways Matthews adhered to this philosophy was in her commitment to the hospital's expansion. Once the new plan was approved, UVMC proceeded with the $42 million renovation, including a new 19-bed, 14,000-square-foot emergency department, an 8-bed intensive care unit, a rooftop helipad, and continually upgraded equipment to meet the current and future needs of patients in the community.

In addition to making sure its infrastructure could handle future demand, the hospital continued to provide a less obvious but equally important contribution in the community: providing hundreds of employment opportunities from entry-level to executive-level positions. According to the California Employment Development Department, wages and salaries for health care in Mendocino County are 50 percent higher than the county average, and the projected growth rate of the jobs through 2018 is twice as high (12 percent) as for other jobs (6 percent). Not only do the health care jobs pay more, they are typically more stable and less cyclical than jobs in many other sectors.

In 2012, the Hospital Council of Northern and Central California commissioned Philip King, PhD, to evaluate the economic impact of hospitals in Northern California. Dr. King's study of Mendocino County indicated that UVMC generated 1,120 jobs and $155 million in spending annually. Construction on the campus expansion project will add an additional 450 jobs and $58.7 million as the project gets underway.

In 2012, UVMC also provided $19 million in charity and unreimbursed care in addition to free health education through its community outreach efforts, including the Children's Health Fair, the Dessert with a Doc program, health screenings, smoking cessation classes, and the Diabetes Education program.

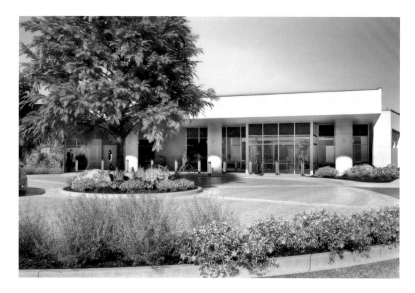

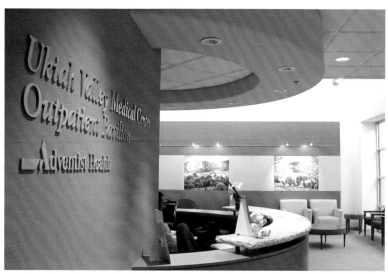

Top: This rendering shows the design of the planned hospital expansion, which broke ground in 2015. Construction is expected to be completed in 2017.

Bottom: Adjacent to Ukiah Valley Medical Center is the Outpatient Pavilion where patients can have labwork and outpatient procedures done. The surgical side is named after Dr. Hugh Curtis, one of Ukiah's most beloved surgeons.

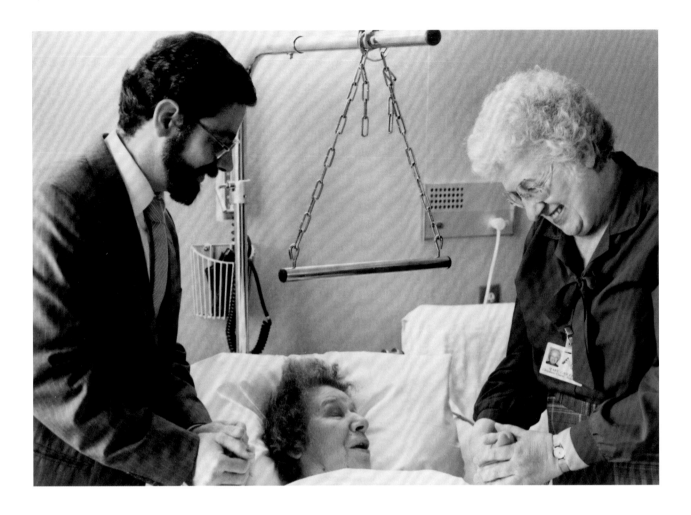

Above: Chaplain Mary Casler (right) offered solace to many patients in accordance with their spiritual beliefs.

Right: To honor her peaceful, supportive, loving spirit, Ukiah Valley Medical Center dedicated Mary's rock.

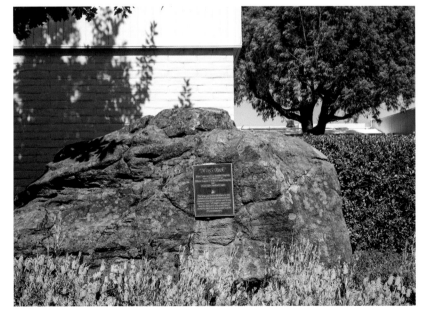

The 2010s represented a critical juncture in Ukiah's health care history: given UVMC's financial losses in the early 2000s and the preponderance of patients who depended on government-sponsored health insurance, as well as the community's depressed socioeconomic status, UVMC's future was none too certain. The Affordable Care Act had passed but had not yet been fully implemented, and it remained to be seen whether UVMC would survive the anticipated decreases in reimbursement.

However, with the help of Matthews' leadership, UVMC was able to fortify community relationships, welcoming collaboration and fostering partnerships with local organizations that promote health and wellness for marginalized populations as well as meeting the needs of employers and the business community.

Matthews says, "In the last few years, UVMC has had the longest steady run of positive bottom line in the history of the hospital, as far back as our records show. Our team has worked relentlessly to keep the life raft of acute care afloat for our community, though we found ourselves navigating through whitewater rapids. We feel that we have been blessed in finding our way."

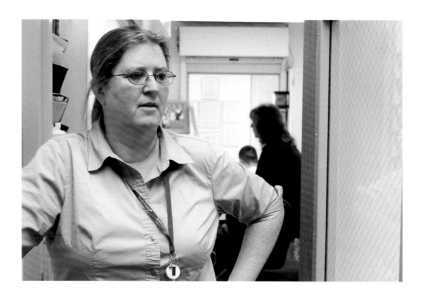

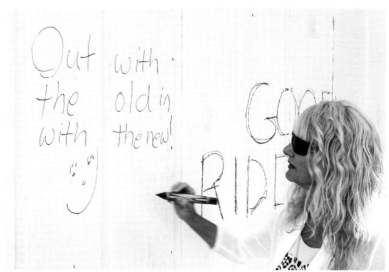

Top: Over many years, Materiels Management Director Kathy Smith earned a reputation as a no-nonsense, get-it-done-without-drama type of person. However, her sentimental side showed when she was offered the hammer to begin the demolition of the Materiels Management building to make room for the new hospital, and she just couldn't bring herself to be a part of destroying her home away from home.

Bottom: Bridget Sholin was one of many employees to write a final farewell to the old building before it was demolished.

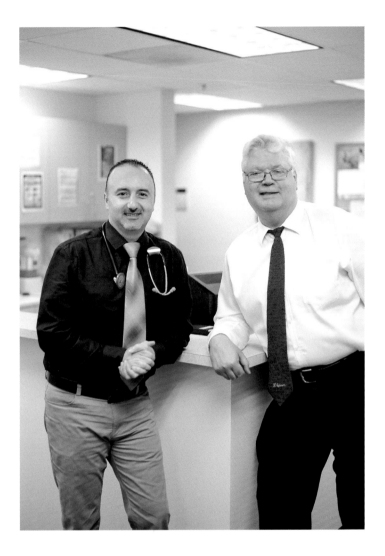

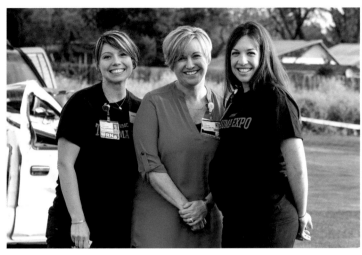

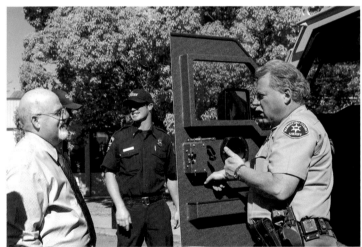

Left: Internist Dr. Iyad Hanna (left) pauses to take a photo with his patient, local real estate broker Dick Selzer, after Selzer's successful treatment of a cardiac condition and sepsis.

Top Right: Registered nurses Rebecca Denoeu, Heather Van Housen and Kristen Marin participate in UVMC's first annual regional trauma expo where dozens of emergency responders watched as the Jaws of Life extricated people from wrecked cars, among other activities.

Bottom Right: Hospital president Terry Burns speaks with Mendocino County Sheriff Tom Allman. The two worked closely together, especially as they sought to improve local mental health resources.

"The quality of life of these people who are in and out of our emergency room has to be improved, and if we don't improve it, nobody's going to improve it. It's up to us."

– Sheriff Tom Allman recalling the words of Terry Burns at the first meeting of the Mustard Seed Coalition

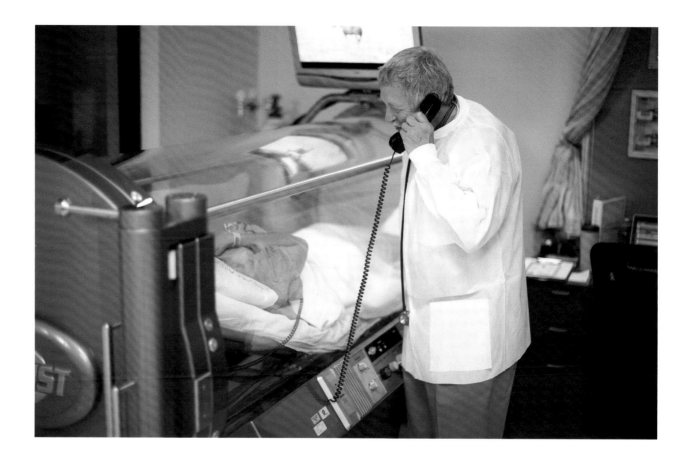

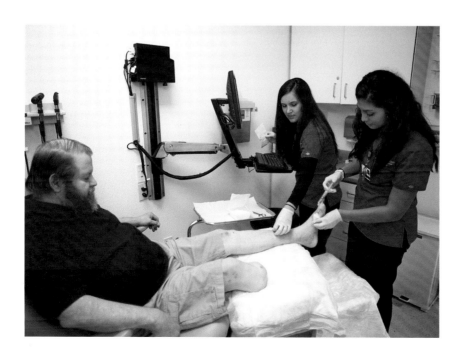

Top: Dr. Fredrick "Tony" Burris talks to a patient in the hyperbaric chamber. This oxygen-saturated environment helps wounds heal more quickly.

Bottom: Wound technicians Rocio Barajas (foreground) and Lacey Rodgers (background) in Ukiah Valley Medical Center's Wound Center help a diabetic patient with his foot care.

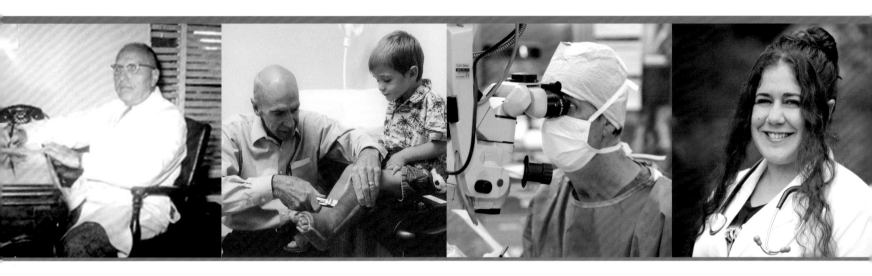

The most important part of the GP's practice was his relationship with his patients. The doctor knew his patients and their families, often personally and professionally, from birth to death.

Doctors

For hundreds of years, small rural towns like Ukiah depended on general practitioners (GPs) and their nurses to provide all manner of medical care. Doctors visited people in their homes to administer care, treating patients in hospitals only when surgery was required, or occasionally to help someone convalesce from a difficult illness. For decades, hospitals were regarded as places to avoid.

Starting in the 1800s, rural hospitals provided a central location for people to receive health care, although it was the doctors, nurses, and other workers in the medical field who made hospitals truly valuable.

Doctors had few tools with which to help their patients. In the early twentieth century, their little black bags might contain painkillers such as morphine and aspirin, quinine to ward off malaria, smallpox vaccine, and digitalis for heart failure.

The causes of many ailments were unknown and often attributed to poor constitutions or degenerate lifestyles, making prevention more difficult until breakthroughs in medical knowledge explained how infection spread.

In the operating room, surgeons asked patients to inhale nitrous oxide or ether for anesthesia, and when performing surgery, surgeons wore aprons over their street clothes to keep the blood from ruining their suits. For years, they wore no gloves or masks, and they sterilized surgical instruments with nothing more than boiling water.

Using only these paltry tools and poor sterilization techniques, doctors were expected to treat ailments such as pneumonia, influenza, and heart disease; stitch wounds back together; birth babies (when midwives were not available); remove gallstones; and perform appendectomies. Doctors could help make people more comfortable and give the body a fighting chance to heal, but until medicine progressed, they could do little more.

Opposite Left: General Practitioner Dr. Jonathan Earl Gardner.

Opposite Center Left: Orthopedic surgeon Dr. Kenneth Hoek removes the cast from patient Jordan Smith's leg.

Opposite Center Right: Opthalmologist Dr. Randall Woesner.

Opposite Right: Family Medicine Practitioner Dr. Miriam "Ida" Harris, who was born and raised in Covelo and returned to care for people in her community.

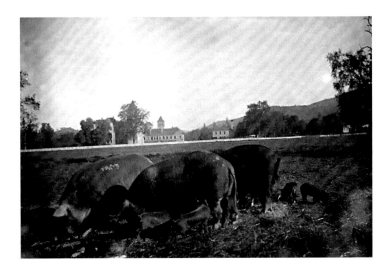

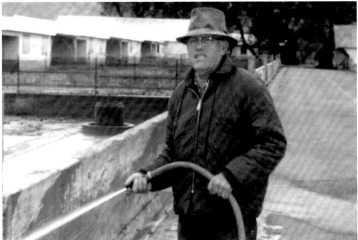

Sunday Drive

Earl Aagaard, grandson of general practitioner Dr. Jonathan Earl Gardner and son of pathologist Dr. Carl Aagaard who helped found Hillside Hospital, recalls visits to the Mendocino State Hospital farm on weekends with his family as a boy in the 1950s and '60s.

> *"We'd pick windfall apples and drink milk straight from the cow. If we were really lucky we'd get to see the piglets," he said. He described stopping on the side of the road to pick grass and feed it to the cows, and the thrill of getting to feed the pigs by throwing food over the edge of the pen. He described watching farm employees feed the pigs with kitchen scraps that were heated with steam to purify them, then pumped out onto a long concrete pad for the pigs. "[The slop] was boiling hot, but as soon as it was on the concrete about fifty pigs would come running," he said.*

Left: Pigs raised at the Mendocino State Hospital.

Right: Walter Freeman cares for the pigs at Mendocino State Hospital.

Dr. Ida May Lathrop-Malpus

A WOMAN AHEAD OF HER TIME

Dr. Ida May Lathrop-Malpus obtained more education than most women of her time. After graduating from Hollister High School in Central California, she attended Florence College. She then went to Miss Field's Seminary (now Mills College) in Oakland and also completed a commercial course at Heald's Business College in San Francisco. In 1897, she graduated from Cooper Medical College (which later became Stanford University Medical School) and then completed two one-year medical internships: one at San Francisco Children's Hospital and one at Santa Barbara Cottage Hospital. Before moving to Ukiah, she worked in San Francisco at McNutt Hospital (later called St. Winifred Hospital).

In 1902, she opened a hospital on the corner of Oak and Stephenson Streets, where she specialized in pediatrics and women's health. In 1909, Lathrop married Al Malpus and chose to hyphenate her surname, which was, like many of her choices, unusual for the era. She was active in civic and social affairs, serving as chairperson of the Ukiah Women's Board for the Panama-Pacific International Exposition in 1915, as secretary of the Mendocino County Medical Association, and as a Worthy Matron in the Casimir Chapter of the Order of the Eastern Star. In her obituary in the *Dispatch Democrat* on June 26, 1931, she was referred to as a "brilliant practitioner."

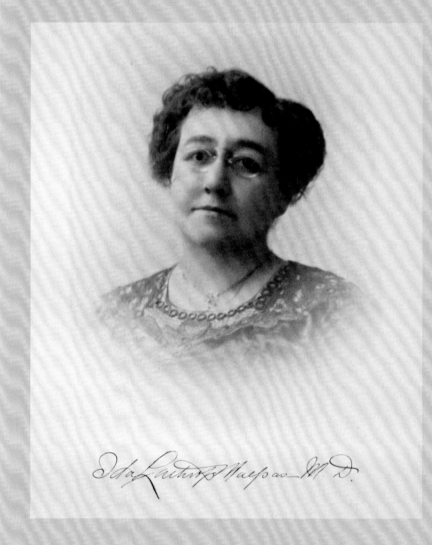

At a time when women rarely became doctors, Dr. Lathrop-Malpus not only practiced medicine, but also founded a hospital. This was one of five hospitals in Ukiah when the entire population was only 1,850.

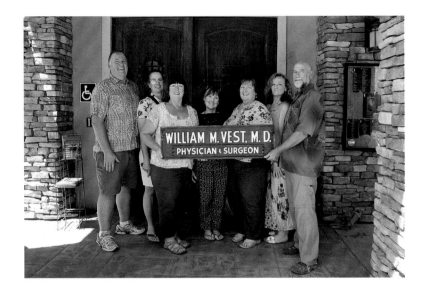

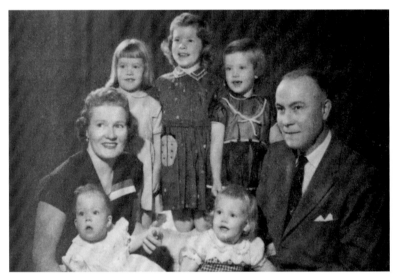

Top: Some of Dr. Vest's children reunite in Ukiah 2016 and hold their father's original office sign.

Bottom: Dr. Wilson was a beloved family physician, pictured here in 1955 with his wife and children.

The most important part of the GP's practice was his relationship with his patients. The doctor knew his patients and their families, often personally and professionally, from birth to death. He cared for kids through playground bumps and bruises, teens through puberty, young women through childbirth, parents through middle age, and grandparents through the trials that come toward the end of life.

When science offered a powerful tool for healing–penicillin–Dr. Jonathan Earl Gardner, a GP who worked in Ukiah in the 1940s, had a mixed reaction. According to his grandson, Earl Aagaard, Dr. Gardner believed "it was a marvelous experience to dispense miracles to sick people for a time. The downside was that a whole different cohort of people began going into medicine. The requirement for someone who could become part of the family of their patients—who could dispense empathy and quiet caring in the many situations where that's all he could offer—that requirement was gone. He wasn't totally sorry; he could do so much more for patients than hold their hands and comfort the survivors, but that part of medicine was important to him, and it pained him to see it passing."

Specialization was rare in the early twentieth century, and female doctors were almost unheard of, making one of Ukiah's early doctors especially notable. Dr. Ida Lathrop-Malpus specialized in the care of women and children and entered Ukiah at the turn of the century. She eventually became recognized by community members and fellow physicians as an outstanding doctor.

For decades after Dr. Malpus' retirement, Ukiah continued to be well served by general practitioners, doctors such as H. O. Cleland, J. E. Gardner, James Massengill, Arthur Miller, Glenn Miller, Walton Joseph "Dr. Joe" Rea, L. K. Van Allen, William Vest, Leland Wilson, and Nicholas

Zbitnoff. They served Ukiah at a time when the local dairy delivered milk to your door, a water truck sprayed the unpaved streets of downtown Ukiah, and house calls were commonplace.

Many GPs cared for patients on a first-come, first-served basis, and patients were willing to wait for hours, if necessary. Ukiah nurse Carolyn Brown, who worked for Dr. William Vest, recalled scheduling appointments only for non-medical visits—if, for example, a businessman needed to speak with the doctor. Tamara Adams said her father, Dr. Zbitnoff, never scheduled appointments, but cared for patients as they arrived. She mentioned that while people waited in his office, they could view the specimens he had floating in jars— among them, her brother's tonsils.

Office hours were simply the hours physicians practiced medicine *from their offices;* working hours were around the clock. After office hours, physicians expected patient calls at home and even unannounced visits from those in need.

Adams, one of Dr. Zbitnoff's five children, recounted being taught from a young age how to answer the phone, "Dr. Zbitnoff's residence," with instructions to find her father no matter where he might be if the caller was a patient. Sally Rea, the youngest of Dr. Rea's six children, also recalled instructions to find her father if someone called, regardless of the time, day or night.

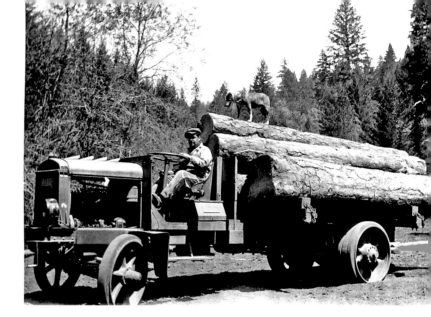

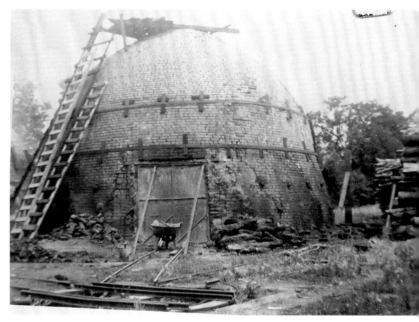

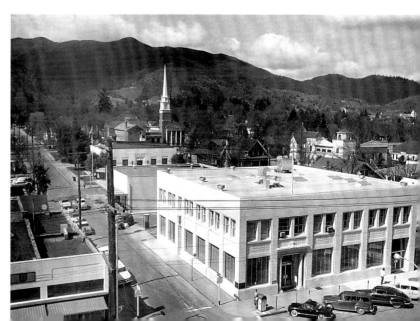

Top: This was typical of the logging trucks carrying old growth redwood logs, circa 1923. Note the dog on top of the logs.

Middle: This kiln, which was run by Goudge, held fifty cords of wood. It took three to four weeks to create charcoal that was then shipped to Hercules Powder Company.

Bottom: Established in 1903, Savings Bank of Mendocino County has been a community cornerstone for more than a hundred years. This building on the corner of School and Standley was remodeled in the mid-1950s to include Ukiah's first drive up window.

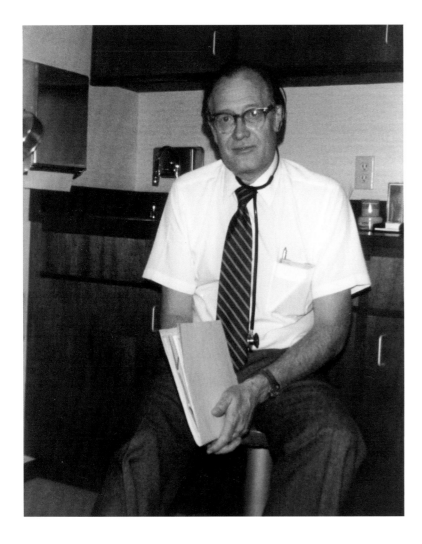

Dr. Eugene "Gene" Lapkass was a beloved general practitioner in Ukiah in the 1960s, beginning his work at the Mendocino State Hospital and eventually taking over Dr. Cloice Biggins' practice.

Brenda Hoek, RN, said she and her fellow nurses used to refer to internists Dr. Walter Bortz, Dr. Gene Lapkass, and Dr. Guy Teran as BLT (like the sandwich)—later BLT and H, adding Dr. Russ Hardy. The internists would visit hospitalized patients together in the morning and then one of them would take emergency call and do evening rounds for all of their combined patients, so the rest could get a break. It was the precursor to today's hospital program.

GPs often brought their children on rounds with them, too. Several of Dr. Vest's six children recalled joining their father on house calls and hospital rounds.

While doctors put in long hours, they did not always get paid in cash (or paid at all). They knew not everyone could afford medical treatment, so they allowed some patients to pay for treatment by trading goods or services. Sometimes, when doctors opted to charge nothing for their care, they would find gifts from patients as expressions of gratitude for their care.

Doctors and their families enjoyed fresh smoked salmon from fishermen, new front doors from carpenters, lugs of peaches from farmers, and sometimes interesting inventions from tinkerers. Before health insurance became commonplace, many doctors balanced their practices so they could afford to deliver some charitable care while still providing a comfortable living for their families.

In 2015, Dr. Michael Turner told a story of finding one of Dr. Eugene Lapkass' old patient receipts (because he had inherited Dr. Lapkass' desk). On the receipt, which was for a total of eleven dollars, the patient had written a note to Dr. Lapkass. Dr. Turner said the note read, "When I broke my leg, you came to Redwood Valley and picked me up and took me to the hospital. Even though I was not your regular patient, you came and saw me in the hospital every day. I think I owe you more than eleven dollars."

While many doctors were willing to treat patients who were cash poor, not all were willing to treat racial minorities. Dr. Zbitnoff opened his practice to everyone.

Dr. Nicholas Zbitnoff

The son of Russian immigrants, Dr. Nicholas Zbitnoff was born in Canada on January 1, 1902. When young Nicholas was eight years old, his father died of an acute appendicitis. A few years later, a kindly pharmacist took the young man under his wing. These events spurred Dr. Zbitnoff's early interest in medicine and eventually led him to serve the Ukiah community as a general practitioner for forty-four years, until he retired at age eighty-three in 1985.

Dr. Zbitnoff chose Ukiah because he wanted to practice in California and Ukiah seemed like a beautiful town, well positioned with a modern hospital. He opened his practice to everyone, including American Indians and other racial minorities, at a time when racial prejudices made non-whites second-class citizens in the eyes of many. Dr. Zbitnoff's ancestry gave him darker skin than some, and he sometimes experienced the very prejudice he did not tolerate in his medical practice.

Dr. Z, as he was usually called, was a lifelong learner with a voracious appetite for knowledge. He was not typically described as warm and friendly—he did not smile too often—but he was deeply interested in people, especially his patients, and he would devote himself to their care with an intensity they appreciated and admired.

Serving as chief of staff at the county hospital as well as running his own private medical practice, Dr. Z was also a father, a gardener, a stamp collector, and a bibliophile with an extensive library. He passed away in 1987, two years after he closed his medical practice.

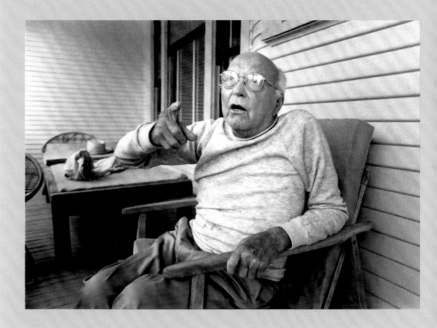

Dr. Nicholas Zbitnoff telling stories on his back porch. Dr. Z, as he was called, was a general practitioner in Ukiah for forty-four years and was still an active practitioner into his early 80s.

Dr. Joseph Rea with two of his daughters Susan (left) and Sally (far right) and his second wife, Irene, dressed for a family celebration in the late 1960s.

Dr. Joseph Rea

A MAN'S TRUE GREATNESS

Dr. Walton Joseph "Dr. Joe" Rea was born in Ukiah on January 26, 1914. The son of a doctor, he grew up in Ukiah, graduated from Ukiah High School, and went on to Stanford University. After receiving his bachelor's degree, he returned to Ukiah and worked as a gas station attendant, among other jobs, but was not particularly enamored with his work. About this time, one of Rea's friends did generations of Ukiahans an enormous favor: he encouraged Rea to follow his dreams and attend medical school.

In 1942, Joe Rea graduated from McGill University School of Medicine in Montreal, Quebec. After serving in the military, he returned to Ukiah and took over his father's general medical practice. In the 1940s and '50s, people said if "Dr. Joe" was not fishing, he was delivering someone's baby. Dr. Rea was friendly and approachable; everyone liked him.

After thirty years of caring for people in Ukiah, Dr. Rea died of lung cancer on March 11, 1976, at age sixty-three. According to his obituary in the *Ukiah Daily Journal*, a friend eulogized him by saying, "A man's true greatness lies in the consciousness of an honest purpose in life, and a steady obedience to the rule which he knows to be right." By that definition, Dr. Rea was a great man.

Until the 1950s, the people who chose medicine as their profession were as varied as the people they cared for, with the exception of sharing a few essential traits. The obvious skills and intelligence required to understand the complex workings of the human body began to filter doctors out of the general public and into a smaller group. A gift for math and science and an interest in helping others were, of course, common. Doctors also had to be willing to deal with issues of life and death. But possibly the single most apparent trait among Ukiah's physicians, both past and present, is their desire to get to the root of a problem and fix it, to be successful detectives and solve the medical mysteries that face them, with or without anyone else's help.

With the arrival of the 1950s came the specialization of medicine. While a GP had been a jack-of-all-trades, medicine began to segment into four main categories: primary medical care, surgery (which later branched into many subspecialties), obstetrics (which sometimes broadened into women's and children's health), and psychiatry.[11]

This trend changed the way people thought about medical care as well as the way physicians related to each other. When faced with an unknown ailment that was causing pain or loss of function, people wanted the very best medical care available, and specialists were assumed to be more knowledgeable than non-specialists. As a result, some of Ukiah's general practitioners decided to go back to school to get more specialized education. Dr. James Massengill became an obstetrician, and Dr. Glenn Miller became an anesthesiologist. These physicians were welcomed back to the community with open arms.

While Dr. Massengill and Dr. Miller were welcomed back to Ukiah after their specialty

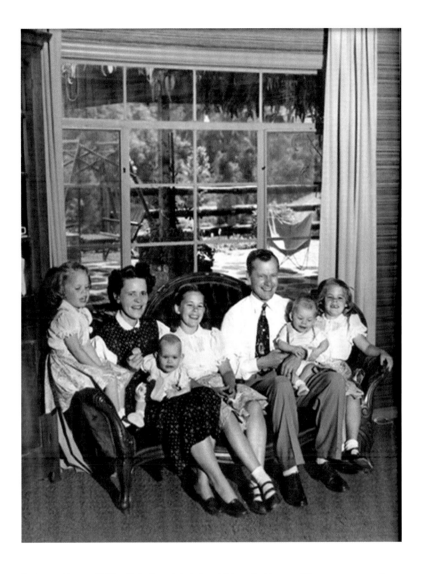

Dr. James Massengill, his wife Josie and their five children. Dr. Massengill began as a general practitioner, but in the early 1960s sought specialty training in obstetrics and gynecology. He returned to Ukiah and practiced as an OB/GYN for the remainder of his career.

Dr. Glenn Miller

FROM GP TO ANESTHESIOLOGIST

Dr. Glenn Miller began his fifty-year career in medicine in Ukiah in 1947, when State Street was State Highway 101 and there were no stoplights in town. He came to Ukiah as a general practitioner to practice medicine with his brother, Arthur. Their wives supported the practice: both nurses, they traded off between caring for their children and serving as nurse to the two physicians.

As one of only six physicians in Ukiah, Dr. Miller had very little free time. During the day, he treated patients from as far south as Cloverdale and as far north as Laytonville, and at night he delivered babies or went to the police station to help officers determine whether someone was legally drunk (in the days before breathalyzers). As many physicians did back then, he made frequent house calls.

By the late 1950s, Dr. Miller's brother had left town to continue his medical studies, leaving Dr. Miller to manage a huge patient load. "The killer was there were so few doctors. I was on call about 100 percent of the time," he was quoted as saying in the Santa Rosa *Press Democrat* newspaper.

After ten years as a GP, Dr. Miller wanted to spend more time with his family, so in 1957 he went back to Loma Linda University Medical School to become an anesthesiologist. He completed his specialty training and stayed to teach at Loma Linda for a short while before returning to Ukiah in 1961. His schedule was more manageable now, and he enjoyed the rest of his career, retiring from anesthesia in 1983 to become director of the hospital's Health Promotion Department.

"There was an altruism about Glenn Miller that you don't see in most doctors—well, that you don't see in most people, doctors or not," said Dr. Donald Coursey, an otolaryngologist who operated with him. "He was a pleasure to work with. He was so calm and easy-going; working with him made cases so much easier."

Dr. Miller was a life-long vegetarian, tennis player, gardener, and advocate for living a healthy lifestyle. He took great pleasure in helping people appreciate the importance of health in all aspects of life—not just physical, but emotional and spiritual, too. He frequently said that life was a great treasure that could not be purchased with any amount of money. In his later years, he wrote a column for the *Ukiah Daily Journal* called "Ask the Doctor," in which he discussed all aspects of health, especially encouraging people to incorporate healthy habits, such as exercise and good nutrition, into their lives. When he visited the hospital, he walked from department to department giving out gardenias, camellias, or whatever was in bloom in his garden.

Dr. Miller passed away in 2015, and his widow, Aldene, ever the nurse, continued to volunteer at the hospital into her nineties.

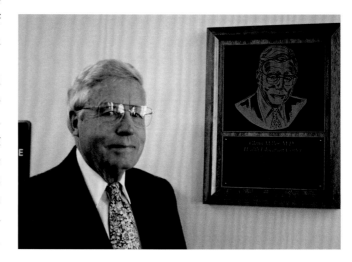

Dr. Glenn Miller in front of the sign bearing his likeness, welcoming people to Ukiah Valley Medical Center's Glenn Miller Conference Room.

training, specialists new to Ukiah were often regarded with suspicion. GPs were concerned that these specialists would threaten their livelihoods. Dr. Robert Werra, who began practicing in Ukiah in 1962, said, "GPs would send tough cases out of town, so no one would know someone more skilled than they were was available locally."

This rivalry almost resulted in one of Ukiah's legendary physicians leaving town because he could not get enough referrals to sustain a general surgery practice (see the following pages for a profile of Dr. Hugh Curtis).

By the 1970s, the number of medical and surgical specialties had grown and the general public often expected to receive the most accurate diagnosis and the most appropriate care from specialists rather than primary care doctors. But until seven of them arrived in Ukiah in the summer of 1976 at Dr. Curtis' encouragement, the town did not have many specialists to offer.

This cohort came to Ukiah to set up medical practices, start their families, and settle into a rural community. They were all men, as the vast majority of physicians were at the time, and their wives typically did not work outside the home; rather, they cared for the home and their children, and actively participated in community events and organizations.

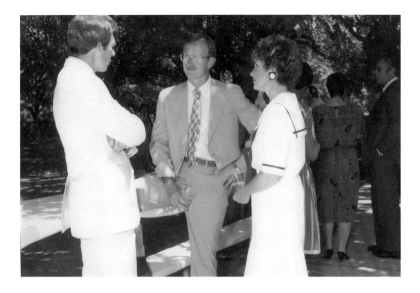

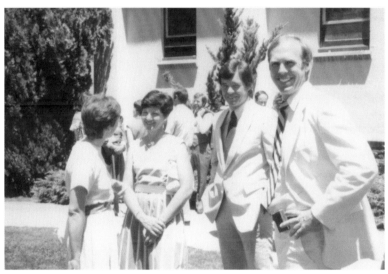

Top: Otolaryngologist Dr. Donald Coursey and his wife Lynda converse with urologist Dr. Robert Blackwelder at a physician event.

Bottom: Urologists Dr. Paul Jepson (right) and Dr. Robert Blackwelder (second from right) smile for the camera while their wives (Pamela and Susan, respectively) converse in the background, circa 1980.

Dr. Hugh Curtis

A SURGEON'S SURGEON

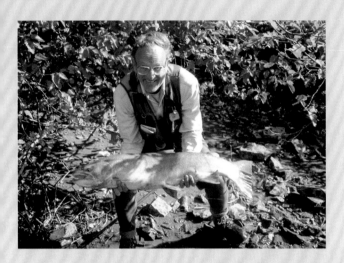

Dr. Hugh Curtis shows off his catch. He enjoyed being outdoors and loved to fish often with his fishing buddy Dr. Joe Rea.

Dr. Hugh Curtis attended medical school at the University of California, San Francisco, and completed his surgical residency at Johns Hopkins University. He passed his boards and went into the United States Army, where he served as the assistant chief of surgery in Landstuhl, Germany, from 1954 to 1957. Dr. Curtis then brought his wife, Phyllis, and their two daughters to live in Ukiah. Dr. Curtis fell in love with Ukiah's natural beauty and rural community, and although he thought the medical community was a little behind the times, he saw wonderful potential.

He worked part-time at Mendocino State Hospital but hoped to build a surgical practice based on local referrals. Before he could begin practicing, however, he had to build an operating room. The operating room at Ukiah General Hospital was so woefully under-equipped that Dr. Curtis felt he could not have performed surgery safely.[12] Thankfully, General Hospital administrator Myrtle Heise agreed to invest in a massive upgrade of instruments and equipment so Dr. Curtis would feel comfortable bringing cases to her hospital.

As Dr. Curtis prepared for a challenging and interesting practice, most local GPs sent the challenging and interesting surgical cases to San Francisco instead of to him. As a result, Dr. Curtis very nearly left for Philadelphia to become a hand specialist under the tutelage of Dr. C. Everett Coop, who later became the United States Surgeon General. In fact, if not for referrals from Dr. Joe Rea (his fishing buddy) and the arrival of Dr. Lee Wilson (a GP, who sent a large volume of patients to him), Dr. Curtis would have had to leave Ukiah.

But the doctor had plans for Ukiah. He was determined to build not only a medical practice but a medical community—and not just any medical community, but one of highly trained physicians who collaborated and continued to learn and grow for their entire careers. He required excellence of himself and those he worked with, bringing specialists from major medical centers to Ukiah to give talks on the most up-to-date medical issues, consulting with experts on difficult cases, and mentoring new physicians who came to practice in the Ukiah area.

Dr. Curtis encouraged internists Dr. Frank Dailey and Dr. Gene Lapkass, otolaryngologist Dr. Matthew Howard, and fellow general surgeon Dr. Bill Fisher—most of whom worked at Mendocino State Hospital—to come to Ukiah. These men joined the handful of physicians practicing in Ukiah, and the nucleus of a modern medical community was formed.

"Hugh had this uncanny ability to recognize extraordinarily capable people and recruit them to help," said general surgeon Dr. Larry Falk, who went into practice with Dr. Curtis in the mid-1980s. "Martin Brotman stands out in my mind. He's one of these guys who, when you're with him for five or ten minutes, you're saying, 'Wait a minute. This guy's a giant.'" Dr. Brotman was a gastroenterologist and administrator at the California Pacific Medical Center (CPMC) in San Francisco. He later became CPMC's CEO and then senior vice president of education, research, and philanthropy for Sutter Health.

"[Dr. Brotman] was a doctor's doctor. Hugh befriended him, and before we had gastroenterologists here, Martin came up to Ukiah and taught us how to do colonoscopies and so forth, extending what we could do here," Dr. Falk said. "So about every two months or so, for years and years, Martin—who is the busiest guy in the world; he's in charge of this multi-billion-dollar hospital—he had so much respect for Ukiah and for Hugh that he would come up, and we'd refer our hardest cases to him. He always had such good suggestions. He was a huge resource, and Hugh was responsible for that."

While Dr. Curtis spent much of his time practicing medicine and building a medical community of dedicated, well-trained physicians, he also enjoyed other pursuits, and everything he did, he did with gusto.

He loved classical music and played the cello, and he loved being outdoors, especially fishing and abalone diving on the Mendocino Coast. Dr. Curtis also enjoyed backpacking, hiking, skiing, and gardening—anything to be outside. While Dr. Curtis was better than most people at managing complicated situations, he also had an enormous capacity for enjoying the simple things in life.

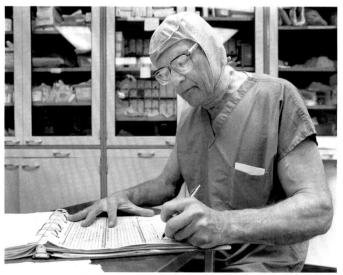

Dr. Hugh Curtis taking post surgical notes.

During his thirty-six years in medicine, Dr. Curtis practiced in a way that inspired colleagues and earned the admiration of patients. When he retired in 1993, he received a letter from Dr. Thomas Russell of California Pacific Medical Center (later the executive director of the American College of Surgeons), who echoed the sentiments of many:

Your style of practice and the depth of your knowledge and enthusiasm for the profession is something that all of us should attempt to emulate. The complexities of your surgical practice far exceed what many of us experienced in a large urban area with the support that we have here. The way your keen mind worked inquiring about new ways to handle a problem was always amazing to me.... You have probably been the most significant factor in medicine in Ukiah for decades.

When Dr. Curtis died on April 12, 2005, at age eighty-one from complications of Parkinson's disease, his widow received more than 250 handwritten condolence cards and letters, many of them pages long. Former patients wrote to share their appreciation for Dr. Curtis' kindness and skill. Colleagues gave their highest praise, saying they would have allowed Dr. Curtis to operate on them any time. Dr. Curtis' obituary said he described his life as a doctor with these words: "It has been a wonderful trip...interesting and fulfilling. I likened each working morning to Christmas.... I could hardly wait to see what the day held."

In recognition of his contributions, Ukiah Valley Medical Center named their outpatient surgery center in his honor later that year.

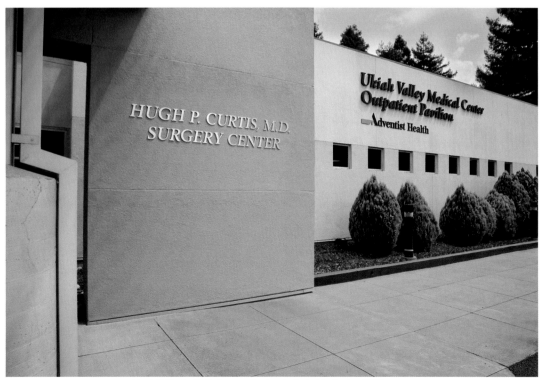

Hugh P. Curtis, M.D. Surgery Center, dedicated in the late 1990s.

The elder statesmen of the medical staff were people such as Dr. Hugh Curtis, Dr. Bill Fisher, Dr. Richard "Dick" Guthrie, Dr. Gene Lapkass, and Dr. Glenn Miller, whose work ethic and quality standards encouraged the new doctors to meet high expectations—which they did. These new doctors, all specialists, were Dr. Albert Baltins, orthopedic surgeon; Dr. Robert Calson, internist and allergist; Dr. David Carter, internist and emergency medicine; Dr. Donald Coursey, otolaryngologist; Dr. Paul Jepson, urologist; Dr. Jack Mason, ophthalmologist; and Dr. Vincent Valente, obstetrician and gynecologist.

One of the reasons physicians such as these were able to settle in Ukiah was because of banker Marty Lombardi. In addition to a decades-long career at the Savings Bank of Mendocino County, Lombardi served as a hospital board member at Ukiah Valley Medical Center. He was known as the "doctors' banker" because of his belief that good doctors were always a good investment.

Dr. Calson reflected on his meeting with Lombardi when he arrived to open his practice in Ukiah. He said he was not quite sure why a banker would loan him so much money given his lack of experience, but he was sure grateful. "Without a loan to get started, I could never have practiced in Ukiah," he said, and he would not have gone on to provide more than thirty years of service as the region's sole allergist, acting as a trusted colleague and cherished doctor.

Many of the doctors who came to Ukiah during the 1970s and '80s were sole practitioners for most of their careers, and they had the autonomy to serve their patients as they saw fit, which typically meant long hours and the rewards that come with being dedicated to one's craft. Most of them got up early, did rounds to check up on hospitalized patients, went to their offices and saw

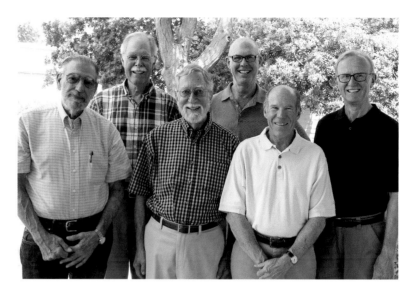

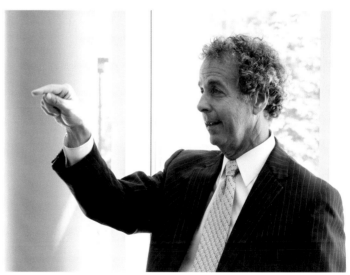

Top: This cohort of specialists arrived in Ukiah in 1976. Front row left to right: OB/GYN Dr. Vincent Valente, ER Internist Dr. David Carter, Ophthalmologist Dr. Jack Mason. Back row left to right: Internist and Allergist Dr. Robert Calson, Urologist Dr. Paul Jepson, Otolaryngologist Dr. Donald Coursey.

Bottom: Banker Marty Lombardi was known as the "doctors' banker." He believed doctors were "a good investment" as he put it, and he was willing to loan them money to support their practices, whether they were just getting started or expanding to serve more patients. Lombardi served on the Ukiah Valley Medical Center Governing Board for many years.

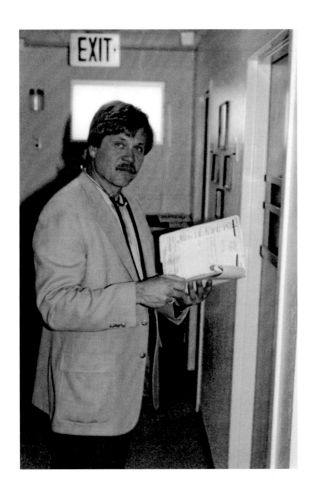

Orthopedic surgeon Dr. Albert Baltins also arrived in 1976, practicing for more than thirty years.

dozens of patients, went back to the hospital to do rounds in the evening, went home for dinner, and then read medical journals until they went to bed. Sometimes they were lucky enough to get a full night's sleep without being called into the emergency room before doing it all again, day after day, year after year. Eventually, these physicians served as mentors to younger physicians, becoming the elder statesmen of the medical staff.

Specialization expanded rapidly in Ukiah—and across the United States—in the decades that followed, and certain personality types were drawn to certain medical specialties, which is still true today.

Primary care doctors are the big-picture people. They enjoy long-term relationships with their patients and are able to connect the dots of emotional and physical symptoms to diagnose health problems, both obvious and subtle.

Dr. Gene Lapkass, one of the most dedicated primary care doctors Ukiah has ever known, said, "We're the chickens of the barnyard. We peck and scratch. We ask, 'How's your sodium? How's your blood pressure?' Not everyone can be a surgeon. They're the eagles that swoop in for the kill and then preen themselves."[13]

Surgeons like to heal with steel. Able to perform well under pressure, surgeons take great satisfaction in a clear and decisive victory: begin the procedure with a tumor, end the procedure without it; go from an ill-functioning body part to a new and improved one, from blockage to clear flow, from a life-threatening wound to beautifully stitched closure.

A Ukiah couple who initially believed their wheezing toddler had asthma discovered it was, to their horror, a cancerous tumor pushing on their son's windpipe. Upon hearing this news, a thoracic surgeon said, "You don't want asthma; that's life-long. We can cut this cancer right out." In this surgeon's mind, a big cancerous tumor was definitely preferable to asthma. He was all about a clear, decisive victory.

Emergency room doctors are the adrenaline seekers of health care. When chaos renders others helpless, ER physicians feel most alive. They are calm and clear-headed under pressure, able to understand and prioritize problems quickly, direct others to assist them, and assure patients that everything that can be done will be done. They thrive on diversity. Internist and ER physician Dr. Marvin Trotter said, "The ER is for us ADD types. We'll do a spinal tap on a seventeen-day-old baby one minute and intubate a seventy-eight-year-old the next."

Psychiatrists choose to work with the body's most complex organ, the mind, determining whether a patient's emotional distress or unusual behavior is a result of a chemical imbalance, a physiological abnormality, or an emotional response to events and experiences in their lives. They are the listeners; they pay attention to what is said and what is not. They pay attention to communication, verbal and non-verbal.

Then there are the doctors who would prefer to deal with the science rather than the patients: the pathologists, radiologists, and anesthesiologists. These are the scientists who often enjoy the mysteries of the body but not necessarily relating to the owners of those bodies. To be fair, though, UVMC has had some incredibly personable and compassionate doctors in these specialties. For example, pathologist Dr. Herschel Gordon went back for additional training to become an oncologist so he could connect directly with patients rather than simply evaluating their tissue samples. He said being an oncologist made him a better pathologist. And when anesthesiologist Dr. Norma Marks discovered one of her pediatric patients, a foster child, was spending his birthday in the hospital, she filled a bag full of gear from his favorite professional baseball team, the San Francisco Giants, and brought it to his birthday celebration.

As with many things, specialization is a double-edged sword. It allows physicians to delve deeply into specific areas of medicine and facilitate some miraculous recoveries, but the growth of specialization also began to fragment health care, changing the doctor-patient relationship into a many-doctors-for-a-single-patient relationship. A GP or family physician, one who had known a patient since birth, had to relinquish

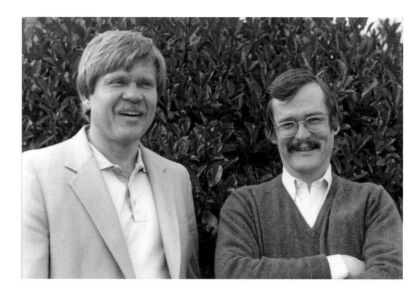

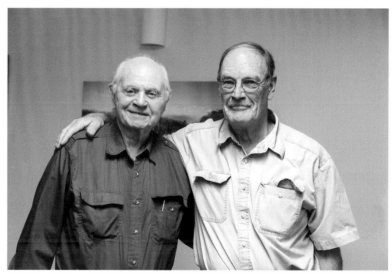

Top: Orthopedic surgeons Dr. Albert Baltins and Dr. Thomas Kilkenny, who practiced in partnership for decades.

Bottom: Pathologist Dr. Herschel Gordon and general surgeon Dr. Larry Falk pose for a photo during Dr. Gordon's retirement celebration in 2015 after four decades of service.

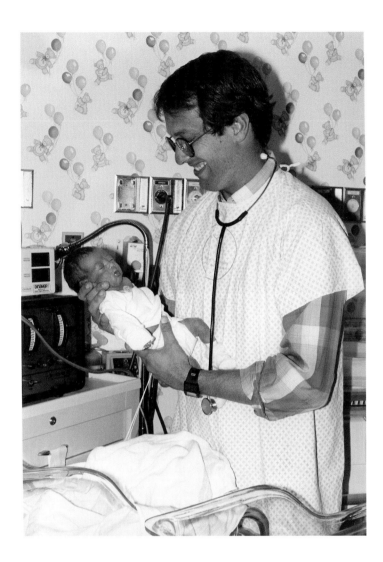

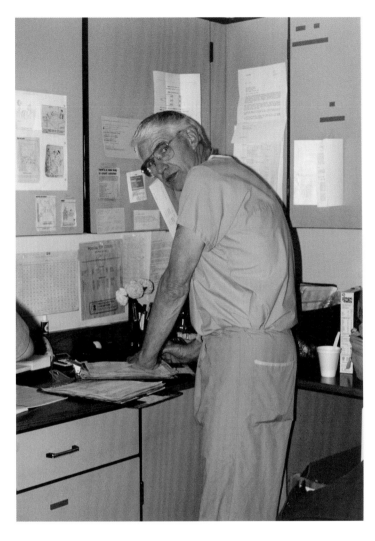

Left: Pediatrician Dr. Richard Miller holds one of the many newborns he saw in the hospital, making sure the babies were healthy and ready to be discharged home.

Right: Pediatrician Dr. Sidney Maurer was known for his unwavering dedication and his excellent care.

Primary care doctors are the big-picture people. They enjoy long-term relationships with their patients and are able to connect the dots of emotional and physical symptoms to diagnose health problems, both obvious and subtle.

his or her patient's care to a specialist who was meeting the patient for the first time. The wise specialist would pay attention to the family physician's assessment and read the patient's medical history, but as Professor Richard Roberts, MD, JD, an internationally recognized leader in family medicine, says, "If you are a hammer, everything begins to look like a nail."

Dr. Roberts commends the excellent work of specialists, recognizing the immense contribution specialization has made to health care. He feels strongly, however, that people should start their care with a primary care doctor; that way, if patients need specialty care, they receive the care appropriate to their condition. It is precisely this type of discernment that primary care doctors are perfectly suited to make because they have long-standing relationships with their patients.

"If you start in the health care system with a specialist, you'll typically get what they have to give. If you have chest pain and you start in a cardiologist's office, you have a high probability of ending up with a cardiac catheterization. Now, that may be what you need, but on the other hand, you may be having stomach acid kicking up into your esophagus causing your chest pain. So, if you happen to start with a gastroenterologist, you might end up with a scope for your chest pain. If you start with an orthopedic surgeon, you might end up with somebody injecting your chest wall for muscle pain. Better to have somebody who knows you as a person, who knows your context, who has a history with you, knows and often cares for your family because these pieces all connect, and that's what family doctors do," Dr. Roberts said.

As medical specialties proliferated, so did the technology to support them, and this, too, fragmented medicine. In the 1950s, before computers, when a doctor needed a second opinion on an

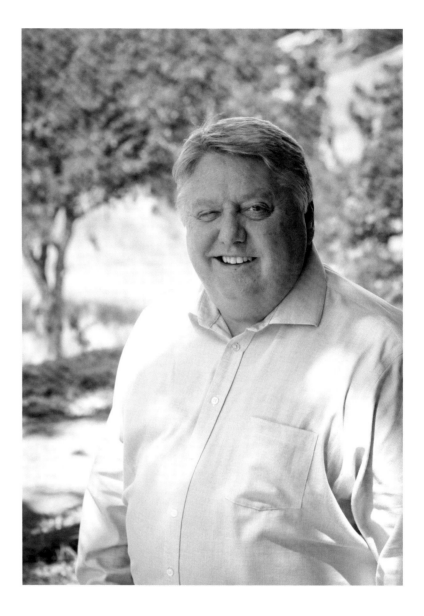

Dr. Richard Roberts visited Ukiah in 2015 and encouraged local health care professionals and community members to pursue their dream of starting a local family medicine residency program.

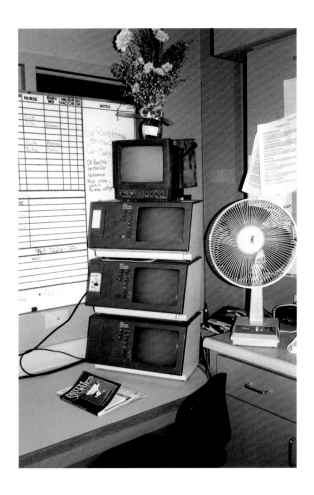

These fetal monitors may look like relics by modern standards, but they allowed obstetricians and obstetrical nurses to hear fetal heartbeats that were undetectable with a stethoscope alone.

X-ray, the X-ray film would be hand delivered to another doctor. When Ukiah GP Dr. Vest wanted to consult with a colleague for a second opinion, his nurse would call Dr. Thomas Nicholson's nurse. The nurses would meet at the back fence to pass the patient's X-ray from one office to the other. The doctors would talk on the phone, and then the nurses would go back to the fence to return the X-ray to its original owner.

Fifty years later, access to X-rays and other radiology studies were instantly available with computers, bypassing the human connection among colleagues. In his book *The Digital Doctor,* author Dr. Robert Wachter of the University of California, San Francisco (UCSF) tells the story of a radiologist whose son invented the Picture Archiving and Communication System for digital transmission of all imaging. The radiologist believed his son had ruined radiology forever because it was no longer necessary for radiologists to share daily dialogue with other physicians who had stopped by their darkrooms to discuss findings. Fortunately, these dialogues still take place daily in Ukiah.

While medical specialization and technology had their downsides, they heralded a new and exciting world of healing. Specialists became true experts in their fields, saving thousands of lives as well as making people whole—restoring vision and the use of limbs, removing cancerous tumors, helping hearts beat steadily, and so much more. Diseases and medical complications that were once written off as hopeless became treatable, even routinely so.

Obstetrical nurse Nyota Wiles shared the story of a Ukiahan who would not have been born if not for the new fetal monitors delivered to the hospital in the early 1980s. A heartbroken pregnant woman was at the hospital to end her pregnancy because her doctor believed her fetus' heart had stopped beating—the pregnancy was no longer viable. An obstetrical nurse eager to try out the new equipment, and always one to hope, suggested using one of the new monitors. The sensitive machine was able to detect the faintest of heartbeats, and the patient and doctor were relieved and elated to have no further need of the hospital's facilities that day. Months later, the woman gave birth to a healthy baby.

With medical breakthroughs providing such amazing results throughout the 1980s and 90s, it is no wonder that specialization, and the technology that supported it, continued to expand.

But while they expanded in the United States, parts of the world remained far behind, lacking even the most basic sanitation, and certainly lacking the equipment and pharmaceuticals to save lives that would have been easily saved in the United States.

Interestingly, Ukiah seems to draw a disproportionately high number of physicians and other health care professionals who have worked abroad at some point in their career. Maybe it is simply that those independent-minded people attracted to practicing medicine in rural Northern California are the same people who are not intimidated by conditions in less developed countries. They are drawn to places where they can make a difference, and if limited resources require creative problem solving, that is okay by them.

Through their experiences on mission trips, the Peace Corps, and others, Ukiah doctors have cared for some of the most vulnerable people on the planet. Many physicians spent months or years abroad, while others took on short-term engagements to heed the call of those facing imminent crises.

General surgeon Dr. Falk said, "This inclination that our medical staff and others in our hospital have to serve overseas is a good thing because it's a healing thread, a connection to something that's deeper than some old prejudices." Dr. Falk led more than twenty medical missions in Guatemala before shifting his focus to Christmas Island, a territory of Australia, inviting medical providers and community members to share their gifts through participation or donations. He noted that mission work is a natural fit for UVMC, as it is a hospital tied to the Seventh-day Adventist church, which has a strong missionary tradition.

Dr. Charlie Evans, chief of staff and director of Ukiah's Pacific Redwood Medical Group in 2015, served as a physician in Kenya before settling in Ukiah. He worked for two years at a clinic that was the only medical facility in a fifty-mile radius and was a two-and-a-half-hour drive away on dirt roads from the nearest hospital. The clinic

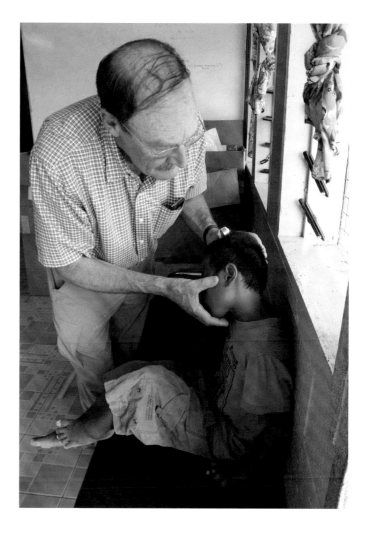

General Surgeon Dr. Larry Falk checked this patient's ear for an obstruction in Guatemala on one of his many mission trips.

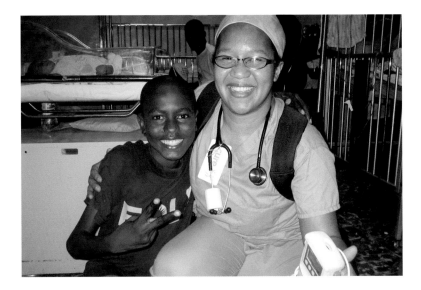

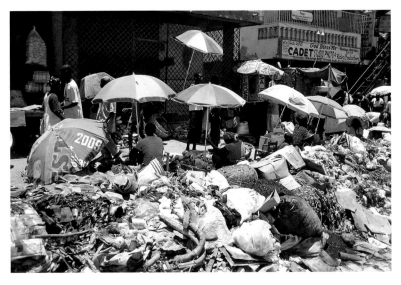

Top: After the devastating earthquake in Haiti, internist Dr. Laura Wedderburn joined many UVMC doctors, mid-level practitioners, nurses, and others on a mission trip. She provided patients with excellent medical care along with her ever-present warmth and compassion.

Bottom: After Haiti's earthquake in 2010, the Haitian medical community begged for international aid. UVMC sent sixty clinician volunteers who helped keep a Port-au-Prince's hospital operational.

was in a small fishing village near Lake Victoria in South Nyanza. It served a broad geographic area of approximately 700,000 people and cared for about a hundred patients a day.

Although the Kenyan clinic had no inpatient beds, the doctors provided all manner of medical care. When Dr. Evans arrived, children were dying of tetanus every week from umbilical cords cut with rusty machetes and the AIDS epidemic was in full swing, but what he remembers the most was how much the physicians did with so few resources.

"To give you an example, when we got there they didn't have a garbage pit—we needed a garbage pit to throw our disposables in. So we built a garbage pit that was six feet deep and six feet high and six feet wide, thinking that when we filled that one we would build another. When we left two years later, we had only an inch of garbage in the bottom," he said.

He explained how they used and reused everything they could. "Every bottle became a vessel for something. Every needle was sharpened and reused. Everything was re-sterilized. You did what you could with what you had." When Dr. Evans returned home, he and his team had left behind almost no garbage; they also left a village with almost no tetanus, polio, measles, or other diseases for which vaccines exist.

Some practitioners who work abroad do so in a time of great need. In 2010, Haiti suffered a catastrophic earthquake, and Haitians requested immediate assistance from anyone willing to help. According to health care provider Lynn Meadows, some major American hospitals (with two thousand patient beds and thousands of employees) declined the invitation to help, explaining that they could not spare any clinical personnel, while UVMC (with only eighty-four beds and a few hundred employees) sent sixty clinician volunteers, who kept a hospital open in Port-au-Prince for six weeks as they took turns serving two-week stints to care for the people of Haiti.

Another Ukiah physician who spent years caring for people overseas is obstetrician and gynecologist Dr. Karen Crabtree, UVMC's Physician of the Year in 2013. Starting in 1989, Dr. Crabtree spent seven years in Malawi, three years in Zambia, and two years in Mozambique. During her time abroad, she provided HIV care and obstetrics and gynecology, and helped to educate midwives. Dr. Crabtree says her work abroad gave her insight into the resilience of women. In Malawi, women do much of the heavy manual labor in their villages, and Dr. Crabtree often needed to persuade female patients to stay in the hospital long enough to heal. Patients did not want to be seen as weak or lazy—so much so that when Dr. Crabtree took a peach-sized tumor out of a patient's bladder, the patient took it with her back to her village to prove she had not been faking her pain to get out of work.

Dr. Crabtree also spent five years in the Navajo Nation in northern Arizona. While the Nation is located within the United States and funded by the Indian Health Service, the people she cared for had very few resources, and they had their own cultural norms with regard to health, birth, and death that differed from the culture of non-Native people.

Whether at home or abroad, doctors in Ukiah tended to run toward challenges rather than away from them. Advancements in science and technology, changes in health care funding, and evolving social norms about individual and community responsibilities influenced how doctors cared for patients. Just as hospitals did, doctors wrestled with how to balance high tech (highly specialized knowledge and treatment) and high touch (relationship-based care), trying to determine when, for example, a specialist's knowledge outweighed a GP's personal connection with a patient, or when the efficiency of retrieving and sharing information via electronic medical records outweighed the ease and familiarity of using paper medical records.

Medical practice in Ukiah shifted again in 1995, this time with the creation of what would become the largest physician medical group in Ukiah's history: Ukiah Valley Primary Care (UVPC). It started as a group with four pediatricians and three family practitioners and eventually became a multi-specialty group with more than thirty medical providers, including surgical specialists, who

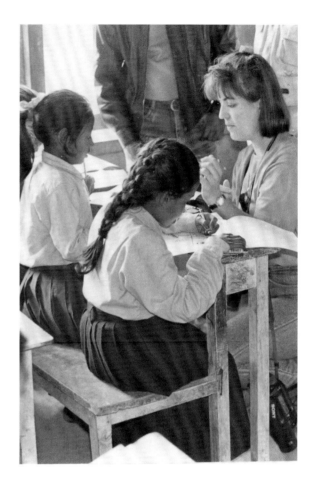

Judy Jutzy, RN, BSN, was one of several Ukiahans who went to a small leper colony outside Kathmandu in Nepal to build additional classrooms for a school in 1995.

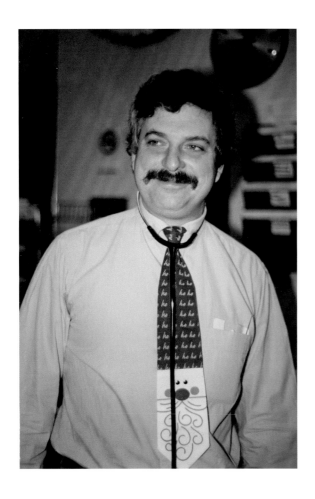

Pediatrician Dr. Jeremy Mann was instrumental in starting Ukiah Valley Primary Care.

cared for a substantial percentage of patients in Ukiah. The original physician members were pediatricians Drs. Connie Caldwell, Samuel Goldberg, Jeremy Mann, and Sidney Maurer and family practitioners Drs. Theron Chan and Robert Werra.

Twenty years on, it is rare to find a solo practitioner. Ukiah's physicians prefer to be employed by one of the groups or clinics in town: Ukiah Valley Primary Care, Mendocino Community Health Clinic, Consolidated Tribal Health Project, Northern California Medical Associates, Pacific Redwood Medical Group (for emergency or hospitalist providers), or the newest multi-specialty physician group in Ukiah, Physician Network Medical Group (PNMG), organized by Adventist Health Physician Services. Many physicians moved from solo practices to groups because of the increasing complexity of medical billing, computer technology, and regulatory requirements; they preferred to focus on patient care and allow someone else to focus on the business side of medicine.

The next twenty years will likely see another shift in the way physicians practice as the Affordable Care Act (ACA) is fully implemented and integrated into American health care. For decades, federal funding has been the driving force behind how medicine is practiced, because federal health care priorities receive the most resources and therefore the most attention.

Going forward, ACA funding encourages doctors and hospitals to work together to put more attention toward wellness and prevention in the hope of keeping patients healthier and thus costs down. Doctors and Ukiah Valley Medical Center will have several opportunities to align their goals more closely. In Ukiah, Physician Network Medical Group represents the foundation model made popular by Kaiser with its Permanente Group. Adventist Health will employ physicians in a medical group, and those physicians will practice in hospitals managed by Adventist Health. This financial model allows Adventist Health (and the plethora of foundations springing up all over California) to continually invest in technology to improve care coordination, health and wellness education and prevention, and case management so patients can avoid having their medical conditions reach the point where they need expensive and possibly invasive health care procedures and treatments.

Another way for physicians and Ukiah Valley Medical Center to work together is through the Mendocino Integrated Care Network

(MICN), a local Accountable Care Organization (ACO). ACOs are groups of doctors, hospitals, and other health care providers who come together voluntarily to provide coordinated, high-quality care to their Medicare patients, according to the Centers for Medicare and Medicaid. A physician can join Mendocino Integrated Care Network as a solo practitioner, a member of a physician group, or an employee of a local clinic. Mendocino Integrated Care Network, supported by Adventist Health, contracts with insurance companies on behalf of its members to establish reimbursement rates for the care of local Medicare patients, and the insurance company then offers incentives for providing excellent quality care, coordinating care, and reducing costs.

Another way doctors and hospitals will work together is through their connection to Partnership HealthPlan of California (PHC). According to the PHC website (www.partnershiphp.org), "PHC is a non-profit, community-based health care organization that contracts with the State to administer Medi-Cal benefits through local care providers to ensure Medi-Cal recipients have access to high-quality, comprehensive, cost-effective health care."

While it is unlikely that medicine will ever support the GP-patient model, it does appear to be shifting back to a primary care model that encourages patients to establish a medical home—a doctor's office or health center—where they go for routine check-ups and the management of both chronic and acute medical problems, only seeking specialty care when referred by their primary care doctor.

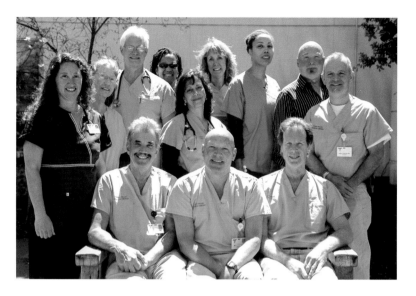

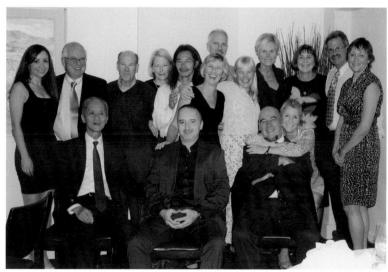

Top: Pacific Redwood Medical Group (PRMG) incorporated in 1993, but members of the group had worked in the Emergency Department dating back to 1981. PRMG started a hospitalist service at Ukiah Valley Medical Center in 2008.

Bottom: Ukiah Valley Primary Care celebrates during the holidays. UVPC began serving patients in Ukiah in 1995.

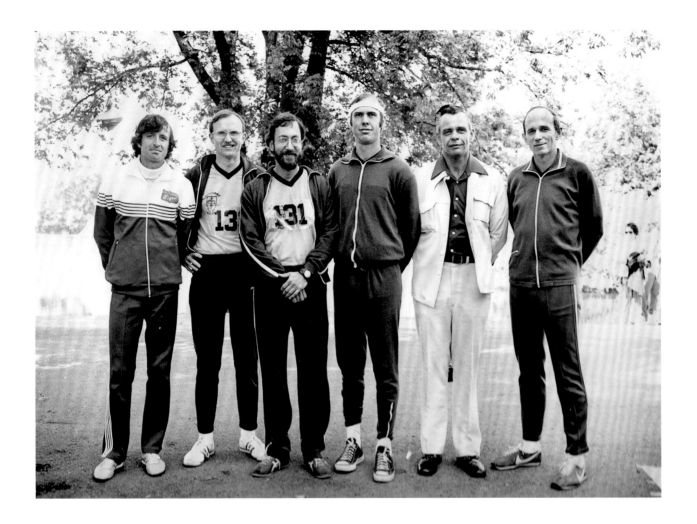

Top: For a few years, physicians participated in the Run for Your Life event. Participants posed with celebrities in the field of health and wellness. From left to right: Olympic 1972 gold medalist Frank Shorter with Ukiah physicians Dr. Donald Coursey, Dr. David Carter, Dr. Paul Jepson, Ukiah General Hospital Administrator Larry Heise, and celebrity doctor Dr. Kenneth Cooper. Dr. Cooper developed the Cooper Method, a way to stay healthy based on an Air Force study using cardio fitness and weight training—basically, the precursor to aerobics.

Right: Run for Your Life participants orthopedist Dr. Robert Kraft who used to run on the defunct railroad in Ukiah by jumping from railroad tie to railroad tie, Dr. Paul Jepson, urologist Dr. Fredrick Graeber, Dr. Donald Coursey.

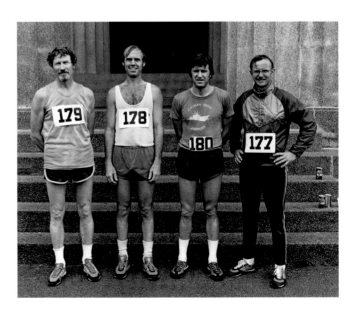

"Run For Your Life"

The HCA sponsored Physicians Relay, an annual event which began last year, will be repeated this year on May 27–28.

This years' team representing Ukiah General Hospital consists of four of our very own great sports, Dr. s Jepson, Coursey, Graeber, and Carter.

This exciting event is an example of HCA's interest in physical fitness for its hospitals, and consistent with HCA's commitment to creating a greater awareness of good health practices.

The Ukiah General Hospital "Team" will be traveling to Nashville for this special event.

We expect to be reading great reports about the outstanding performance of the Ukiah General Hospital Team ! ! ! You show them how it's done Doc's ! ! ! Good Luck.

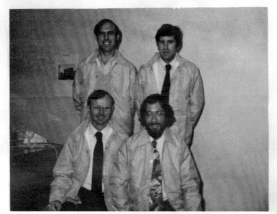

"At The Finish Line"

Pictured "at the finish line" are each of the Ukiah General Hospital Relay Team Members whom we all know and love ! ! You'll all swell with pride to know that out of 35 teams participating in the 1977 H.C.A. Annual Physician's Relay, the U.G.H. Team placed 12th ! !

Dr. Jepson (upper right) added to it by placing FIRST in his heat ! . . . . . We're Sooo . . . . . proud of you Doc's ! ! !

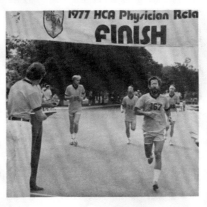

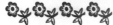

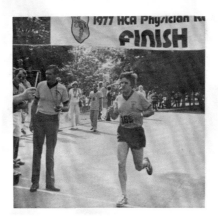

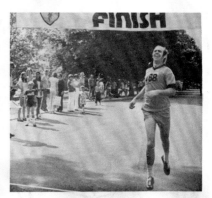

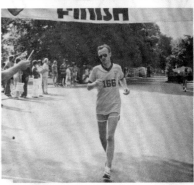

"The HCA sponsored Physicians Relay, an annual event which began last year, will be repeated this year on May 27-28…. The Ukiah General Hospital 'Team' will be traveling to Nashville for this special event."

Newspaper coverage of the Run for Your Life event.

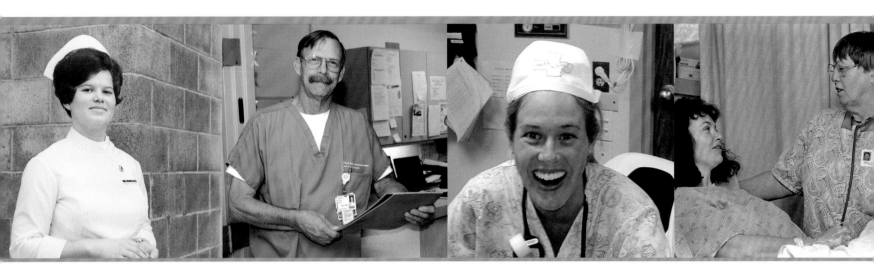

Nurses are more likely to ask how they can help rather than how they can be helped. And while nursing has changed dramatically since its inception, the people drawn to the profession have not. At its core, nursing is still about connecting with people when they are vulnerable and helping them feel better.

Nurses

Since people have been on the planet, they have nursed each other back to health or provided comfort when health could not be restored. In many societies, long before modern doctors and formal medical schools, healers and wise women passed on knowledge from generation to generation to help those with ailing minds and bodies. These were some of our first nurses.

Through the years of modern medicine, doctors would have had a difficult time caring for patients the way they have without help from nurses.

People drawn to nursing are fulfilled by helping others. Nurses are typically caring and compassionate, often detail-oriented and solution-based in their thinking. Successful nurses are good communicators, which means they express themselves well and, perhaps more importantly, are patient, attentive listeners. Nurses are more likely to ask how they can help rather than how they can be helped. And while nursing has changed dramatically since its inception, the people drawn to the profession have not. At its core, nursing is still about connecting with people when they are vulnerable and helping them feel better.

Two nineteenth-century nurses who helped establish the profession were Florence Nightingale and Clara Barton. During the Crimean War, Nightingale and a team of nurses improved the unsanitary conditions at a British base hospital, reducing the death count by two-thirds, and Nightingale's writings sparked worldwide health care reform. Barton was a hospital nurse during the American Civil War who went on to establish the American Red Cross. From these early traditions, nursing care flourished.

In large part, nursing in the United States evolved along the same path as medicine. Originally, nursing care required no special training and nurses learned what they needed to know on the job, either from other nurses or from the doctors who employed

Opposite Left: Shortly after graduating from nursing school in 1969, Sue Jutten, RN, served as a nurse at Hillside Community Hospital. In 2016, she works in the same building as a nurse for Mendocino Community Health Clinic.

Opposite Center Left: Cecil Gowan, RN, has worked as a nurse at Ukiah Valley Medical Center for more than twenty years.

Opposite Center Right: When the hospital was short-staffed, it would bring in traveling nurses like this one.

Opposite Right: Nina Curtis, RN, cares for a patient.

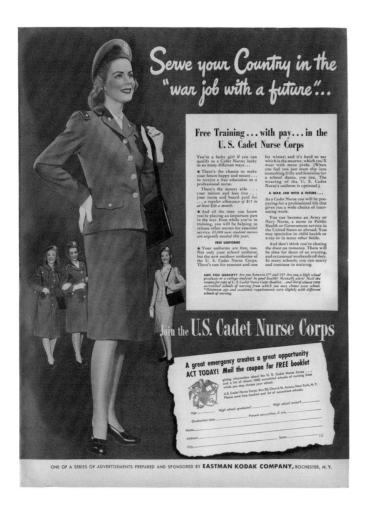

Above: Ads like this encouraged young women to contribute to the war effort by becoming nurses.

Opposite: The surgery theater at the Mendocino State Hospital was state-of-the-art when it was built. On the left is the head surgical nurse, Carmen Lucchesi, and her assistant preparing for an upcoming procedure.

them. All nurses were generalists, or "practical" nurses. But as medical knowledge expanded, treatments and procedures grew increasingly complex and doctors needed assistance from nurses with more skill and education.

In the early 1900s, the Rockefeller Foundation funded the Goldmark Report, which identified gaps in nursing education and helped lay the groundwork to create strict standards for nursing schools. In 1923, Yale University was the first collegiate school of nursing to adopt the Goldmark Report standards. The Rockefeller Foundation led to the formalization and standardization of university-level nursing education.[14]

In the first half of the twentieth century, careers for women were limited; basically, women could choose either nursing or teaching. Those who chose nursing were immediately recognizable by their uniforms—white caps with their school's insignia, white dresses, white stockings, and white shoes. When they went outside on a cold day, they wore heavy wool nursing capes, navy blue with a red lining. Surgical nurse Dorothy Bowen, who worked at Hillside Hospital from its earliest days, said those wool capes were "heavy as the dickens."

Throughout the early part of the century, nursing students worked twelve-hour or even twenty-four-hour shifts, providing cheap labor for many hospitals. Because nursing traditionally meant long hours, relatively low pay, and nurses were viewed as doctors' handmaidens, the profession did not attract as many nurses as the country needed. This became especially problematic as the United States went to war in the 1940s.

In fact, according to the American Association for the History of Nursing, "extraordinary measures were necessary to meet the increased demand for nurses during World War II." On July 1, 1943, Congress passed the Bolton Act, establishing the United States Cadet Nurse Corps and providing funding to train more nurses. More than 85 percent of the nation's 1,300 nursing schools participated, graduating 124,065 nurses between July 1, 1943, and June 30, 1948.[15] One such nurse was Ukiah's Carolyn

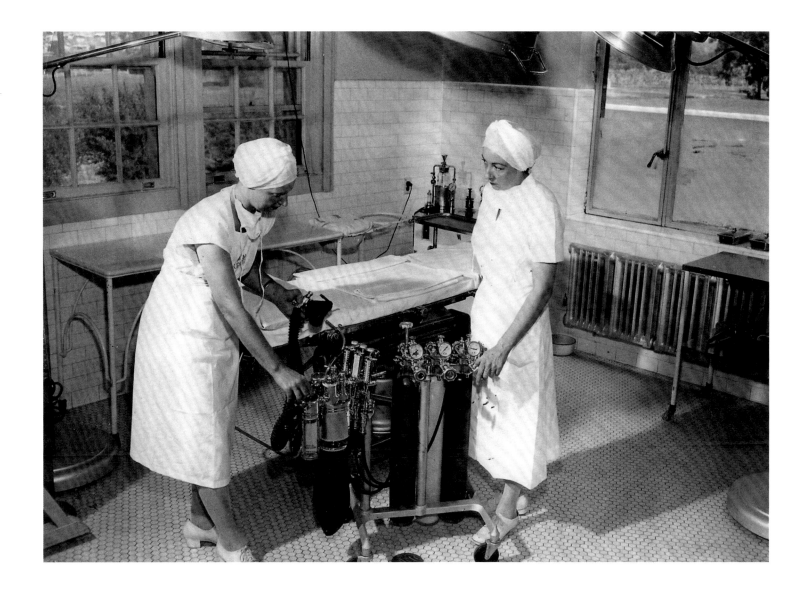

Those who chose nursing were immediately recognizable by their uniforms—white caps with their school's insignia, white dresses, white stockings, and white shoes.

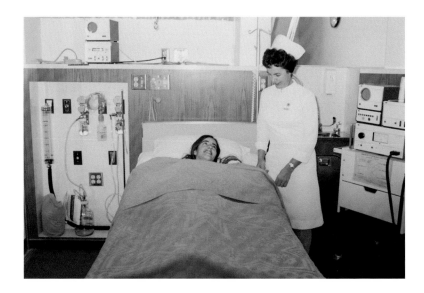

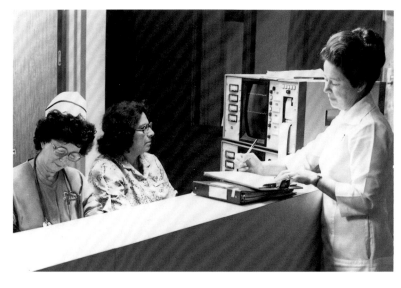

Top: In the early 1970s, nurses continued to wear whites and the nursing caps that identified their nursing school.

Bottom: Electronic monitors allowed nurses to keep track of several patients simultaneously from the nurses station. Pictured left to right: Lillian Pacini, RN, Gladys Devine, RN, and Jennie Ward, LVN.

Ford (now Carolyn Brown), who attended nursing school at Mills College in the San Francisco Bay Area from 1943 to 1946.

"They needed nurses so badly that they paid our way through nurses' training during World War II. I was in the first class. When I got out of high school, I was just-turned eighteen, and by July 12, I was at Mills College taking all these classes—psychiatry, pharmacology, nutrition, anatomy and physiology, and all this stuff. And we lived on the campus—we lived in Mills Hall," Brown said.

As nurse training was a military program, strict rules applied. Brown mentioned, for example, that the nursing students in the cadet program were not allowed to date enlisted men, "only cadets or officers."

"I would have gone into the Army as a second lieutenant or the Navy as an ensign if the war was still on, but it wasn't. I was sent to Albuquerque, New Mexico, to the veteran's hospital," she said. "It was an experience. It was horrible when the soldiers came back." She paused, thinking back, then explained how some soldiers returned home with tuberculosis and other ailments. "They made these boys fight even with all these diseases."

After her service, Brown moved home to Ukiah. She recalled being a brand new registered nurse in 1946, working nights at Ukiah General Hospital. "You worked twelve-hour shifts, six days a week, and I think they paid me $172.00 per month. I had one nurses' aide who was sixty-eight, and she only worked eight hours [a day]; four hours she was sleeping at the hospital. And here I was at twenty-one years old—emergency room, maternity room, everything. And they didn't write orders; nothing was written, but the nurses knew the doctors so well that they knew what the doctors wanted. Well, I was new, and I came from a strict school of nursing where everything had to be just so, but here—no orders." She lasted about two months before leaving to work in a hospital in Oakland. It would be years before she returned to work as a nurse in Ukiah.

In the 1950s, the nurse's scope of practice began to expand, following the path that the doctors had trail-blazed when they became specialists. Surgeons needed nurses with specialized knowledge to support them. Hospitals needed nurses who specialized in each type of care: emergency care, intensive care, labor and delivery, pediatrics, and more. Nurses began to focus their studies on the elements of medicine that interested them most.

Although nursing modernized, it was a far cry from today's norms. In the 1950s, syringes were still made of glass and had reusable needles. IV bags did not exist; rather, glass IV bottles were used, and doctors (not nurses) took a patient's blood pressure and hung IVs because such work was considered above the level appropriate for nursing. Blood pressure information was not shared with patients for fear of upsetting them, and there was no such thing as cardiopulmonary resuscitation (CPR). Finally, if a patient's behavior was out of control, it was up to the discretion of the nurse whether to use patient restraints, which were made of leather and none too comfortable.[16]

As nurses gained training that allowed them to provide higher levels of care, patients still needed practical nurses and someone to help with the bathing and bedpans. Associate nursing degree programs sprang up in community colleges, which helped reduce the cost of the education, and nurses' aides were trained in vocational schools or on the job.

In the 1960s and '70s, the first baby boomers entered nursing; they were the largest cohort ever to enter the profession, and they helped move nursing from a temporary vocation to be left in favor of marriage and motherhood to an academically grounded, life-long profession.[17]

Even though the 1970s gave rise to the women's equality movement and inspired nurses to ask for better pay and better working conditions, when doctors arrived at

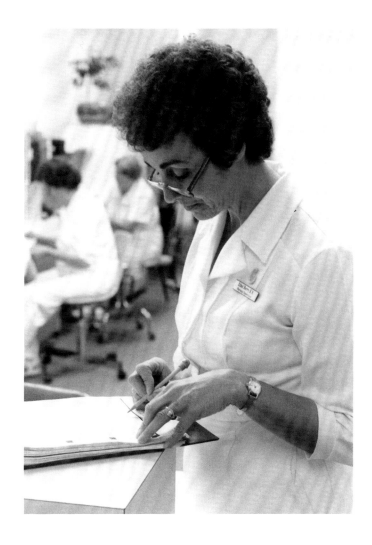

Ethel Berry, RN, reviews a patient's chart. Berry later became an inspector for the California Department of Health Services, reviewing hospitals in Mendocino, Lake, and Sonoma Counties.

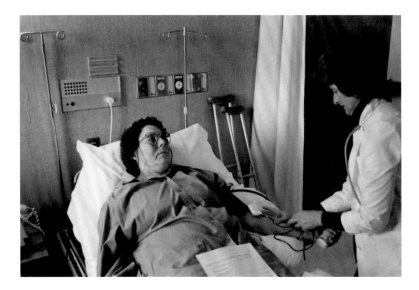

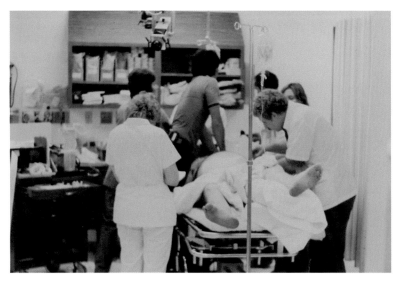

Top: As the nursing profession developed, doctors depended on nurses to take vitals, monitor patients and start IVs.

Bottom: In the Emergency Department, nurses have to remain calm, even in the face of chaos.

Opposite: This 1971 nurse graduation ceremony shows the overwhelming number of women as opposed to men who went into the profession.

the nursing station, nurses were still expected to stand and offer their seat to the doctor and to hand over the patient's medical chart, even if they were not finished with it.

Nurses carried a Kardex everywhere they went: a large, folded card on which they documented patient activities and medications; it was hand-written in pencil so it could be erased and updated as needed. Patients were addressed as Mr. or Mrs., and nurses wore gloves only for sterile procedures, because they worried that patients would misinterpret the wearing of gloves to imply they thought the patients were somehow dirty. Medicine was dispensed by a nurse who carried a tray with small paper cups of pills and different colored med cards.[18]

Ann Johnson, RN, former emergency department nurse and founder of Wild Iris Medical Education, said gloves did not become commonplace in Ukiah until the 1980s. "We didn't wear gloves until AIDS. No one did," she said.

Through the 1970s and '80s, the nurse's role continued to evolve. Increasing levels of specialization and responsibility led to the introduction of "Nursing Diagnoses," the nationwide shift that depended on a nurse's clinical judgment about a patient's condition and its potential to cause other health issues and medical complications.

The American Nurses Association notes that a nursing diagnosis reflects not only that the patient is in pain, for example, but also that the pain may cause other problems, such as anxiety, poor nutrition, or conflict within the family, or has the potential to cause complications. The nursing diagnosis is the basis for the modern-day nurse's care plan.[19]

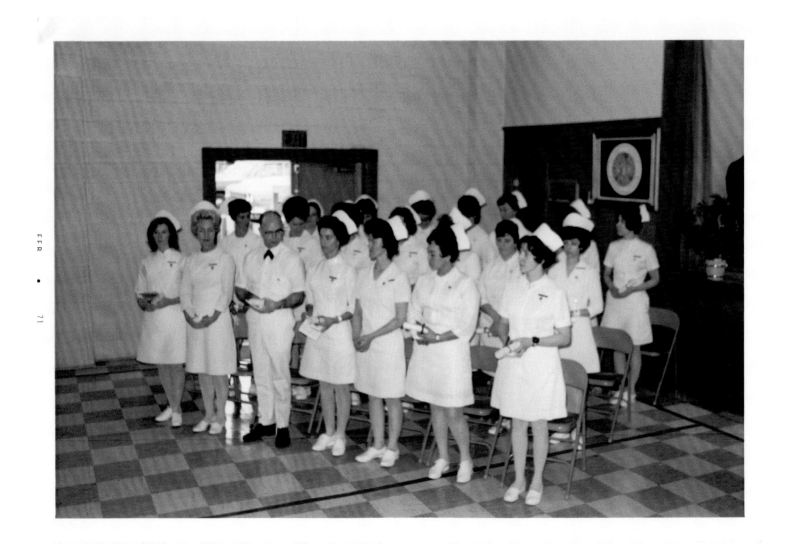

*Originally, nursing care required no special training and nurses
learned what they needed to know on the job.... All nurses were
generalists, or "practical" nurses. But as medical knowledge expanded,
treatments and procedures grew increasingly complex and doctors
needed assistance from nurses with more skill and education.*

Candy Gorbenko in 1971, a recently graduated registered nurse.

Candy Gorbenko, RN

FORTY YEARS A SURGICAL NURSE

Candy Gorbenko grew up in Ukiah, a dentist's daughter who once passed out watching her father extract a tooth. If you had asked her whether she would grow up to be a surgical nurse whom doctors admired and held up as their favorite, she would have answered a most resounding, "No chance!"

When she finished high school, Gorbenko's parents recommended pursuing an education that would allow her to support herself financially, so she completed a two-year registered nursing program in 1971. She began working as an RN on the night shift in the intensive care unit at Hillside Hospital and said she "hated every minute."

Recognizing her unhappiness, the surgical nurse manager, Dorothy Bowen, RN, offered to teach Gorbenko basic sterile technique and have her help out with cases in the operating room, after which Gorbenko's opinion of nursing began to shift.

Shortly thereafter, Gorbenko got married, and she and her husband, Mike, moved to Glendale so her husband could finish his studies. When Gorbenko sought a nursing job at Glendale Adventist Hospital, she was able to land a job in the operating room (OR), where she remained for the next four years. In the 1970s, at large facilities like Glendale, nurses were specializing in more than just surgery—they became surgical specialists like their physician counterparts. Gorbenko worked primarily as an otolaryngology nurse (specializing in ear, nose, and throat surgery).

In March 1975, the Gorbenkos returned to Ukiah and were due to have their first baby in August. Candy was hired back at Hillside Hospital on a contingent basis and, during the next five years, was able to keep up her skills in the operating room while caring for her children.

As with physicians, nurses gravitated to areas that best suited their personalities. Shy by nature, Gorbenko liked the controlled atmosphere of the operating room rather than dealing with floor nursing "where patients were awake," she said with a knowing smile. As her three children grew and more hours became available in the operating room, she eventually began working full time.

She loved working in a small-town operating room, as opposed to the one in Glendale, because, she said, the surgeons were different. "Anybody coming to a small town has a different mentality. They aren't so wrapped up in their practices that they can't enjoy life. And I think we, as nurses, feel we spoil our physicians. We protect them. I think doctors do know [we take special care of them], even if they don't verbalize it. We're kind of a family," she said, describing how they share life's ups and downs and often spend time together outside of work.

Gorbenko said nurses in big-city operating rooms demand their breaks, expect to finish their shifts on time, take vacations when it is convenient for them, and get pigeonholed into narrow specialties. "In Ukiah, we have fewer people, so we cover each other's backs," she said, citing examples of trading vacation time when it helps a colleague or finishing a case rather than having the next nursing crew finish it. "It's better for patient care. Working in the OR takes an emotional toll. Experience helps you get through it, plus the rapport with the doctors," she said.

She related stories about cases that have stayed with her through almost forty years of nursing: helping Dr. Laurie Spence save a young man's life—he had barely missed severing his carotid artery when barbed wire cut his neck during an all-terrain vehicle accident; working with Dr. William Bowen through the night for ten hours straight while he worked on every limb of a patient who had been in an automobile accident; working with Dr. Donald Coursey while he reconstructed the face of a young man who had tried to commit suicide by shooting himself.

The volume of instruments and equipment in the OR has grown tremendously. From high-tech implants to specialized microscopes, technology continually provides new and better ways to help patients live longer, more comfortable lives—and surgical nurses must learn what each of these things is and does so they can support the surgeons who use them.

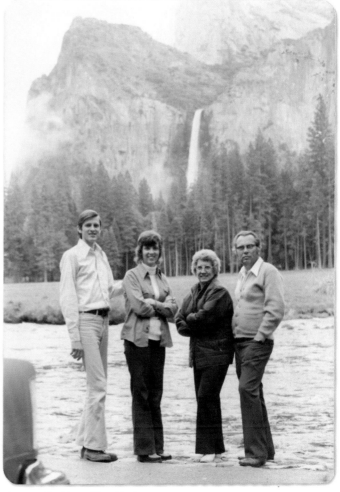

Candy Gorbenko with her husband Mike (left) and parents Patricia and Donal Anderson.

According to Gorbenko, the technology that most transformed the OR was video, because every member of the team could see what was happening in the surgical field. Gorbenko said once she could see what was going on, she could often predict what a surgeon would need by watching his or her progress on the video screen, making the whole process more efficient.

Retired nurse Aldene Miller told a story that her husband, anesthesiologist Dr. Glenn Miller, shared with her. "Candy is such a good scrub nurse. Glenn said the surgeon would put his hand out for the next instrument, and before he could say what he needed, she had it in his hand."

Video also opened up the world of laparoscopic surgery, allowing surgeons to make small incisions and use flexible tubes to insert air into a patient's abdomen or use balloon dilation in the sinuses, and then perform surgery with much faster recovery times because the procedures are so much less invasive.

Gorbenko talked about her appreciation for the skill of so many of the surgeons she has worked with. "I love Dr. Coursey's dressings, and Dr. [Ziad] Hanna is just awesome to watch," she said.

While Gorbenko believes the culture of the OR has not changed much since she began as a nurse, she said health care is more egalitarian than it used to be. In the OR, a clear chain of command keeps patients safe, but as long as everyone is respectful, all members of the surgical team are encouraged to speak up. "We gain the trust of the doctors over time," she said, adding that she feels completely comfortable sharing any concerns she has with the surgeons she assists.

All these years later, Gorbenko is glad she became a nurse, but maybe not half as glad as the surgeons she has worked with. Dr. Larry Falk described her as "priceless" in the operating room, adding, "Candy is a beautiful combination of competent and affable. She's mature. She knows what she's doing. She's a pleasure to work with."

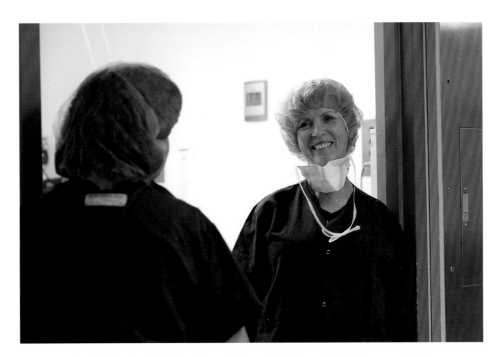

Candy Gorbenko (right) talks with anesthesiologist Dr. Norma Marks before a case in 2016.

Outside of the operating room, some nurses continued their studies until they became mid-level providers. In the 1970s, the University of California at Davis used funding from a Johnson & Johnson grant to spearhead a rural bridge program, training capable registered nurses to become nurse practitioners (NPs). NPs were medical providers in their own right, able to prescribe medication and provide treatment that used to be solely in the realm of the physician.

As the program was about to begin, UC Davis had two nurses from Covelo, one from Mt. Shasta, one from Etna, and one last slot to fill. UC Davis' program director, Dr. Hughes Andrus, approached family physician Dr. Robert Werra in Ukiah to see if he would be interested in participating in the program, which meant selecting a registered nurse to become an NP, mentoring her as a preceptor, and then hiring her once she successfully completed the program.

Dr. Werra chose ICU RN Jean Quinones, who eagerly jumped at the opportunity. Each week, Quinones boarded a plane sent by UC Davis to Ukiah's small municipal airport to transport her to classes at UC Davis, which she attended Monday through Wednesday. Thursdays and Fridays she spent in Dr. Werra's office. When she completed the program, Dr. Werra offered her a ten-year contract to work with him as a private nurse practitioner, one of the first in Ukiah.

The popularity of working as a mid-level medical provider grew, and eventually multiple paths to the profession emerged. Many mid-level providers came up through the ranks of the registered nurses; others attended school to become physician assistants after completing a pre-med undergraduate education. The most common mid-levels are nurse practitioners, physician assistants, certified registered nurse anesthetists, and certified nurse midwives.

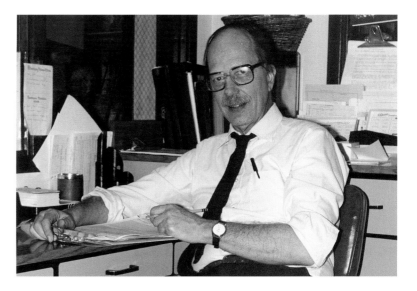

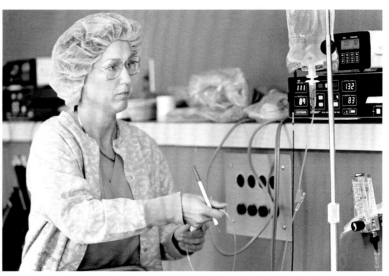

Top: Family Medicine Practitioner Dr. Robert Werra was named the California Family Physician of the Year in 2005.

Bottom: Nurses continued to take on increasingly complex responsibilities. JoAnn Beck, RN, prepares for surgery.

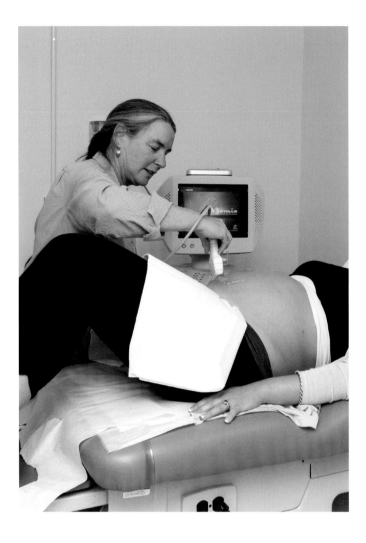

Certified Nurse Midwife Maria Finnegan uses ultrasound to assess the health of the fetus.

In a 2015 interview, obstetrician and gynecologist Dr. Karen Crabtree said she was heartened by the shift in health care funding that encouraged health care professionals (from nurses to technicians to mid-levels) to work to the top of their licensure. Having worked in a health care system inspired by a European model, she believed in a team approach and saw first-hand the effectiveness of allowing mid-level providers to offer most primary care, using specialists only for cases that require that level of knowledge and skill. Dr. Crabtree felt mid-level providers could offer some specialty care, too, depending on the specialty—for example, certified nurse midwives managing prenatal care and births unless a complication arose.

"I think midwives do the best care for women because they have the time and that's what they are trained to do. They are very focused toward midwifery, whereas a lot of doctors come out of medical school and, while they might end up going into a certain specialty, [midwifery] wasn't something that motivated them from the beginning," Dr. Crabtree said.

As patients began to play a larger role in their own medical decision-making, nurses progressed from patient caregivers to caregivers *and* advocates. Nurses worked with patients and their families to help determine whether a patient was physically and mentally capable of making informed decisions about care and treatment, and then took on the role of health educators, sharing information with patients so they could make medical decisions effectively.[20]

The 1980s brought the end of nursing caps, the shift from nursing whites to more comfortable—and practical—scrubs, and the introduction of more men into the field. Educational opportunities expanded and nursing licensure became stricter, including the requirement that nurses pass the NCLEX test (national nursing boards). According to registered nurse Ann Johnson, California demanded higher scores than other states, and the two-day test covered all areas of nursing specialties: positioning, pediatrics, medical/surgical, medication, orthopedics, coronary, pulmonary, obstetrics, and more.

Lynn Meadows, PA

REBEL WITH A CAUSE

In Ukiah in the 1970s, as with most everywhere in America at that time, when it came time for women to deliver babies, they were rarely asked before they were catheterized, shaved, given an enema, and their feet were placed in stirrups. Women were sometimes tied to their beds, and when they did not progress quickly enough for the attending physician, they received Pitocin to speed the birthing process along. Midwives were not considered medical practitioners, and water births were unthinkable.

This is when a young, idealistic lay midwife named Lynn Meadows moved to Greenfield Ranch, a communal-living, back-to-the-land paradise just outside Ukiah, where organic food and self-sufficiency were the order of the day and rejecting mainstream values was commonplace.

Meadows and other local midwives, such as husband-and-wife team Ross and Linnea Ritter, recognized that many young women wanted a more natural childbirth experience than the one offered at the hospital, so they began a birth center, "which was nothing more than an office where we would meet and talk with women," Meadows said. A small group of lay midwives worked together, with the private support of some local physicians, to help women give birth at home. Even after being sued by a local obstetrician who feared Meadows was putting patients at risk, Meadows did not stop. Eventually, these midwives helped the medical establishment recognize the value of a more natural process, which was then adopted at local hospitals.

After becoming a physician assistant and working in Mexico for a year to become bilingual in Spanish, Meadows joined Pacific Redwood Medical Group and began working in the UVMC emergency department, where she remained until 2009, when she transferred to the hospitalist service. This move is what ignited her interest in palliative care.

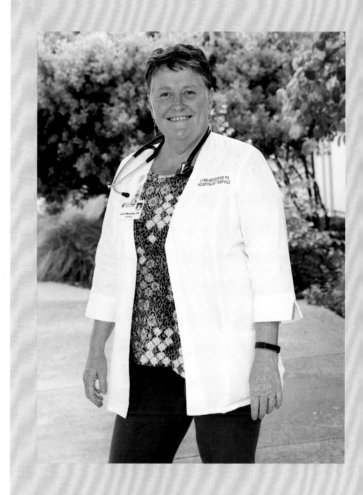

Physician Assistant Lynn Meadows now leads the Palliative Care team at Ukiah Valley Medical Center.

The next year, Haiti suffered a catastrophic earthquake, and Meadows was one of the sixty volunteers from Ukiah who boarded a plane and flew to Haiti to care for victims in Port-au-Prince, with the secondary goal of supporting an orphanage.

Already a poverty-stricken country suffering from human trafficking and child slavery, Haiti crumbled under the devastating earthquake. The basic infrastructure required to facilitate recovery was decimated, and morgues were overrun with more than 100,000 dead.

Meadows was among those from Ukiah who discovered the Reveil Matinal Orphanage and vowed the orphanage's twenty orphan girls would not be lost in the rubble. She and others committed their love and determination to assure these girls would be kept safe and receive an education. They founded Hearthstone Village, and in 2016, seven years (and seven more girls) later, it was going strong.

As a result of her humanitarian efforts overseas, Meadows' attitude toward mitigating pain and suffering evolved, so much so that she shifted her professional focus at home to become the leader of the hospital's palliative care team.

According to Dr. Marvin Trotter, who worked with her for years in the ER, Meadows is a "powerhouse in a small package." At not much more than five feet tall, her energy and enthusiasm as well as her confidence that seemingly insurmountable challenges are pebbles to be knocked aside, make her the perfect person to lead in uncharted territory.

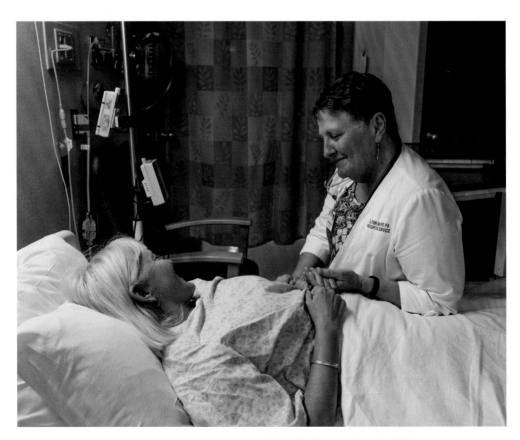

Lynn Meadows takes time to speak with patients and their families when the end of life is near.

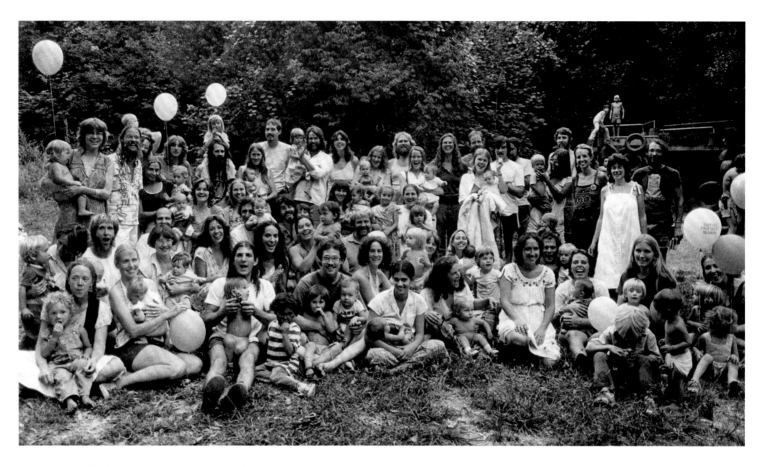

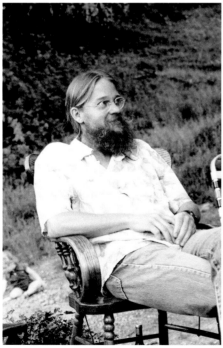

Top: Lynn Meadows was part of the Birth Center in the 1970s and '80s, a group of like-minded people who felt modern medicine was too intrusive during the birthing process. This photograph was taken during a fundraiser. The Birth Center offered classes and prenatal care across the street from the old Palace Hotel.

Left: Ross Ritter (pictured) and his wife Linnea were instrumental in helping women have a more natural birthing experience.

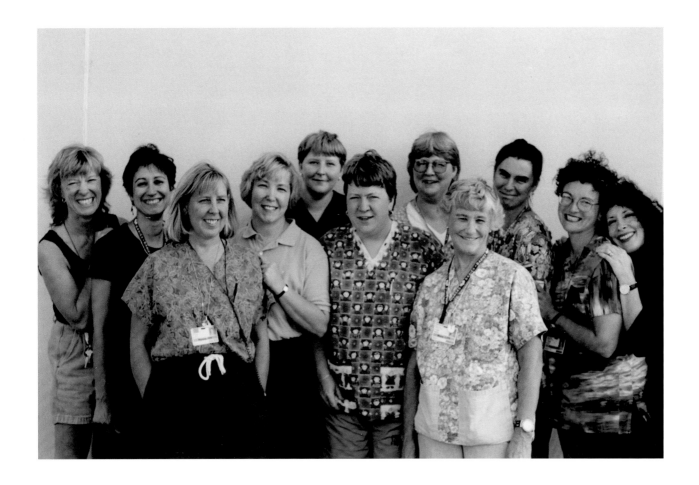

Top: Obstetric nurses pour their care and love into each newborn. Left to right: registered nurses Nancy Bray, Sofia Costas-Smith, Nyota Wiles, Carolynn Wyatt, Heidi Chaney, Linda Dashiell, Laura Roberts, Mary Denna, Mary Swensen, Karen Wilson, and perinatal educator Isa Davila.

Right: Proud parents Adina Merenlender and Kerry Heise show off their son, Noah, born April 27, 1998, the first baby born in the new obstetric facility.

Opposite: To address the national nursing shortage, Ukiahans took matters into their own hands and created a nursing program at Mendocino College.

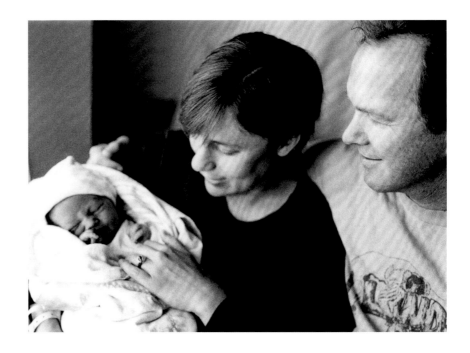

Nursing knowledge and skills continued to grow and expand in the 1990s. Many more nurses had become mid-level providers, and some specialized further, becoming family nurse practitioners, pediatric nurse practitioners, certified registered nurse anesthetists, and certified nurse midwives. While they continued to work with physician oversight, they practiced with tremendous autonomy.

As a nationwide nursing shortage emerged during the 1990s, it was clear that Ukiah would have trouble recruiting and even maintaining its nursing ranks, because UVMC could not compete with the financial resources of competing hospitals. Understanding their strong position, nurses in California led a nationwide trend to demand higher wages, more generous benefits, and better working conditions through organized labor. Some Ukiah nurses wanted to join the California Nurses Association, but Ukiah Valley Medical Center's status as a religious not-for-profit organization helped make it exempt from labor unions. Elements of unionization were inconsistent with Adventist beliefs. The hospital did, however, raise salaries and improve benefits, both because they recognized the value of their nurses and because they did not want to lose qualified nurses to competitors. Though this helped retention, it did not solve the shortage. Once again, people in Ukiah faced a national problem and came up with a local solution.

MENDOCINO COLLEGE NURSING PROGRAM

UVMC chief nursing executive Jerry Chaney had the foresight to understand the value of a local nursing program and had long advocated for the development of a nursing program at the local community college, Mendocino College. However, new programs require new funding, and nursing programs require expensive clinical facilities; the college did not have the capital (financial or political) to develop a program.

In 1999, Dan Jenkins, a former public health nurse with a history of developing innovative programs such

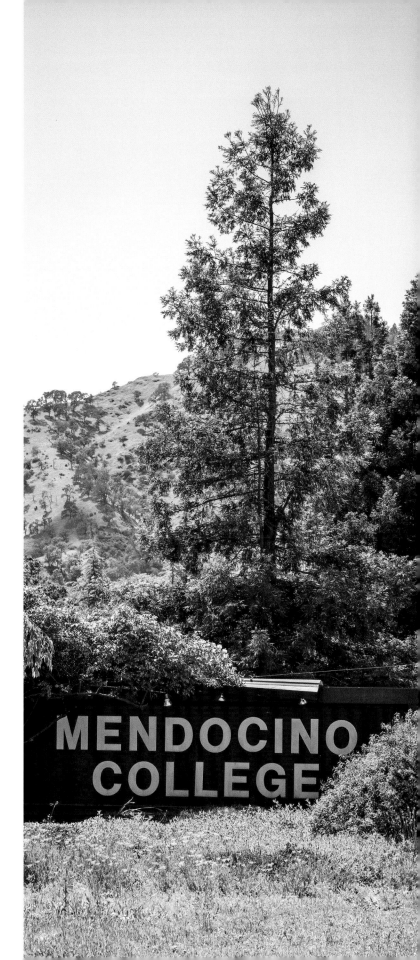

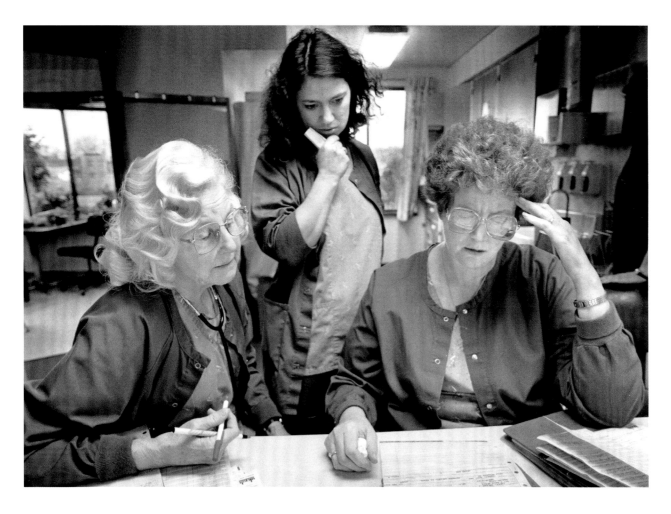

Top: Left to right: registered nurses Luella Case, Cindy Stacy, Judy Hennigan collaborate to assess the best course of action.

Right: Nurses and volunteers take a moment to pose for a photo before going back to their busy days.

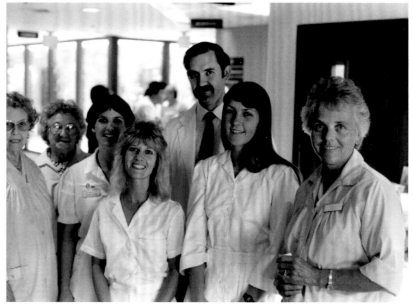

as the highly successful Drug Court, became Mendocino College's director of Health and Human Services programs. When Chaney approached him about the need for a nursing program, Jenkins immediately began the complex process of garnering approval for a new college program, including undertaking a labor market study and a community needs assessment. Jenkins simultaneously began developing curriculum as well as facility and program designs to meet the Board of Registered Nurses' strict requirements.

In 2003, the LVN-to-RN bridge program was approved by the Mendocino College chancellor's office and accredited by the California Board of Registered Nursing. This allowed licensed vocational nurses to become registered nurses, but the community still did not have a start-to-finish nursing program.

The California Board of Registered Nursing required Mendocino College to employ a program director and an assistant director for an accredited program. Jenkins knew the college did not have funding for the positions, so he approached local hospitals to see if they could help. Frank R. Howard Memorial Hospital in Willits immediately stepped forward with financial assistance, and the college was able to hire Barbara French as director and Fran Laughton as assistant director. These women were responsible for developing the full registered nursing program.

Jenkins lauded the roles of both Jerry Chaney, whom he called "really instrumental" in the development of the nursing program, and the public health officer at the time, Dr. Marvin Trotter, who enthusiastically supported the program. Jenkins also shared his appreciation for the nursing directors at all the local hospitals who participated in the steering committee and helped develop the program.

On Chaney's advice, UVMC President Terry Burns asked Jenkins for a pro forma to determine the cost of starting and maintaining a comprehensive nurse education program. Burns then offered to fund the lion's share of the program, committing $60,000 per year indefinitely, and asked Howard Memorial Hospital in Willits and Sutter Lakeside Hospital in Lakeport to each fund $20,000 per year. Blending this funding with student tuition and support from the college allowed the program to get underway.

Today, Mendocino College offers both a two-year registered nursing program and an LVN-to-RN bridge program. Completing the program leads to eligibility for licensure as a registered nurse.

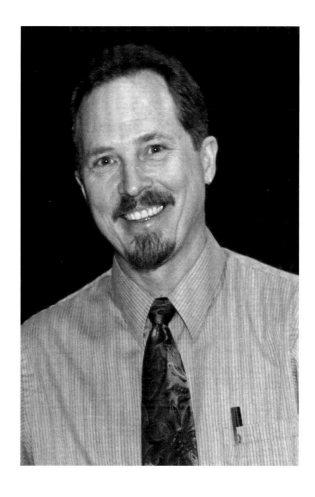

Mendocino College faculty member Daniel Jenkins was instrumental in creating the nursing program at Mendocino College.

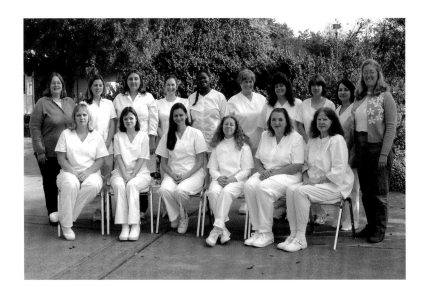

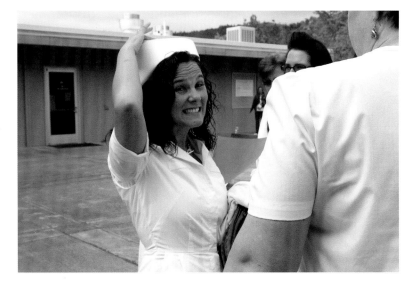

Top: In 2004, Mendocino College graduated its first class of registered nurses. The fourteen graduates are flanked by their primary instructors, Dr. Barbara French (left) and Fran Laughton (right).

Bottom: Jene Lowater celebrates the conclusion of her program at Mendocino College in 2007.

Upon completion, the graduate receives an associate degree in nursing and is eligible to sit for the California State Board of Registered Nursing licensing exam. The program boasts a pass rate of 100 percent on the licensing exam, in large part thanks to Al Beltrami, a community member who honored his wife's memory by supporting one of her passions: education.

Beltrami was the county administrator from 1964 to 1989, and when his wife, Pat, passed away, he decided to donate part of her estate to the Mendocino College Nursing Program, specifically to pay for all new nursing graduates to take their boards immediately after completion of the program, while their knowledge is fresh. This key piece of financial support allowed new nurses to become licensed so they could immediately enter the workforce and put their hard-earned knowledge to good use.

The associate degree program is a full-time two-year program that offers a series of courses that combines academic classes on campus, skills practice in the nursing skills laboratory, and patient care experience in various hospitals and facilities, primarily in Mendocino County and Lake County.

To generate interest in health care careers such as nursing, Ukiah Valley Medical Center helped establish the Scrubs class at Ukiah High School and provides opportunities for young people to shadow health care professionals during their workday.

Jerry Chaney, RN

A LIFE OF SERVICE

Registered nurse Jerry Chaney has always been known for his willingness to collaborate and his gentle way of helping others make difficult decisions with grace and wisdom. He leads by example and patiently works toward goals that—to his way of thinking—must be taken care of by someone, and that might as well be him.

Chaney graduated from nursing school in 1969 and began working nights on the medical/surgical wing at Hillside Hospital in March 1971. "Within the first couple of days, a patient coded," Chaney said, explaining his trial by fire when a patient stopped breathing. Because there was rarely more than one registered nurse working during a shift—and licensed vocational nurses and certified nurse assistants were not allowed to provide certain types of care—the registered nurse's responsibilities could feel overwhelming to a new nurse. Chaney rose to the occasion and was quickly promoted.

During his first year, he became the PM-shift charge nurse, and then he moved to the emergency department, where he became the nurse manager. When Chaney began his nursing career in Ukiah, Hillside Hospital had only one ER bed, but soon added four more as a result of an agreement between Ukiah General Hospital and Hillside Hospital to divide care in Ukiah: General would provide obstetrics, and Hillside would provide emergency care.

In 1975, Hillside Hospital began offering Ukiah's first emergency care with a dedicated on-site doctor twenty-four hours a day, seven days a week. In 1974, the Mendocino State Hospital closed, and Hillside Hospital's ER was inundated with mentally ill patients who had nowhere else to go, a problem that continues today.

Unlike today, doctors in the early 1970s shared city call (being available to come in at a moment's notice to provide hospital emergency care), whether they were dermatologists, pediatricians, or surgeons. If an accident or illness was outside a physician's comfort zone, he would call a colleague. "Everyone wanted friends

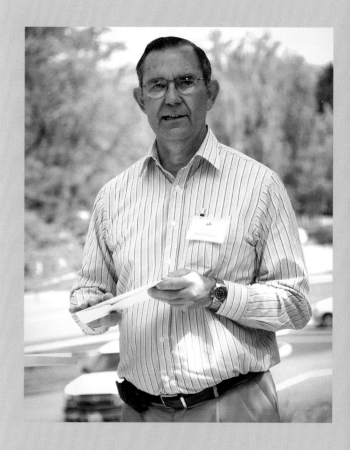

Jerry Chaney, RN, has served as a model nurse, nursing administrator, and board member for local non-profit organizations. He is a quiet force who continues to address health needs in the region.

to come to their aid, so everyone came when called," Chaney said.

Chaney continued as the ER nurse manager for years, helping to build the new hospital facility on Hospital Drive (and finding out first-hand how well his friends in the ER took care of people when he required stitches after a mishap with a chainsaw while clearing pear trees for the new hospital site).

A year after Ukiah Adventist Hospital purchased the assets of Ukiah General Hospital in 1988, it was renamed Ukiah Valley Medical Center (UVMC). In typical Chaney fashion, though he belonged to the Seventh-day Adventist Church, he saw the original name as divisive and successfully led the petition resulting in the change to UVMC.

People who have worked with Chaney use words like gentle, thoughtful, thorough, and capable to describe him. And one of Ukiah's most successful medical businesses, Pacific Redwood Medical Group (PRMG), was inspired to create a corporate culture based on Chaney's open communication and willingness to share work fairly. "Many aspects of Jerry's work as the ER nurse manager helped set the tone for PRMG," said Dr. Ron Gester, one of PRMG's founders.

Chaney's influence continued to grow, and in 1984 he became the hospital's vice president for patient care. It was in this role that he helped others in health care and in the community at large to recognize the threat of the nursing shortage in Ukiah. He not only worked with local leaders in education to advocate for a local nursing program, he also advocated for licensed vocational nursing and certified nursing assistant programs through the Ukiah Unified School District Adult School.

Chaney resigned from UVMC in 2001 and went to work as the chief operating officer at Mendocino Community Health Clinic. In 2005, he became the chief nursing officer at Healdsburg District Hospital before returning to UVMC to reprise his role as vice president of patient care in 2007. He retired in 2012 but maintained his role as an influential health care leader through his participation on non-profit boards for the Mendocino College Foundation and Mendocino Community Health Clinic.

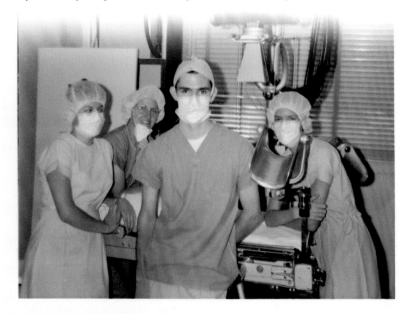

Jerry Chaney, RN, pictured early in his career, circa 1971.

The nurse who followed in Chaney's footsteps as the hospital's vice president for patient care was Heather Van Housen, a registered nurse whose dedication serves as an example for even the most seasoned nurses. Van Housen has held many nursing roles, from floor nurse to nursing instructor to risk manager. Once she was appointed as the hospital's chief nursing officer, she implemented a daily safety call that occurs at 0800 every morning. Nurse managers from every department participate, and even if Van Housen is not on campus, she calls in. "It doesn't matter where she is on the planet," UVMC president Gwen Matthews said, "even when she's on vacation. It's like clockwork; she's on that call making sure all safety issues have been taken care of and any new concerns are identified and addressed."

Like doctors, nurses have expanded their scope of practice and specialized during the past sixty years. As one of very few professions initially considered appropriate for women, nursing has evolved as attitudes toward women have evolved in this country, from a doctor's lowly assistant to a respected health care professional. According to a Huffington Post article by Charles Tifin, PhD, published in March 2013, today's nurses (men and women) are "giving TED talks, publishing scientific research, developing mobile medical applications, and actively addressing health care policy."[21]

Matthews said, "Nursing provides a deep understanding about the complex operations of patient care and all that it takes to support it, and that provides a strong base for health care leadership, as evidenced by how many administrators in Ukiah have been women who were nurses." In Ukiah in 2016, two of the top hospital executives are both women and registered nurses.

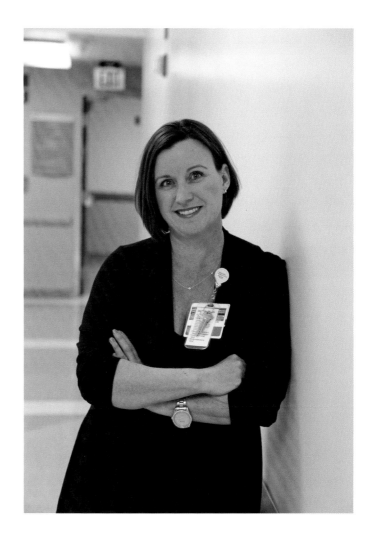

Ukiah Valley Medical Center Vice President of Patient Care Heather Van Housen followed in Jerry Chaney's footsteps, providing dedicated and compassionate leadership.

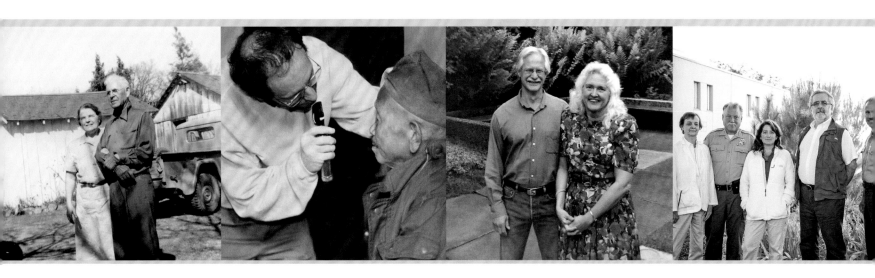

Truly, one of public health's greatest challenges—and achievements—has been to address not only disease, but also the health disparities caused by poverty, prejudice, and other barriers.

Community Care

Opposite Left: Dr. H. O. Cleland with his second wife Ida. Dr. Cleland served as Mendocino County public health officer for decades.

Opposite Center Left: Defining "community" broadly, Ukiah physicians participated in mission trips to remote parts of the world. Pictured: Dr. Geoff Rice examines a Nepalese man's eye.

Opposite Center Right: Dr. Marvin Trotter with Carol Mordhorst in the 1990s. At that time, Dr. Trotter was the Mendocino County Public Health officer and Carol Mordhorst was the Public Health administrator.

Opposite Right: Health care providers and members of law enforcement worked together to address mental health problems.

While the health of individuals in Ukiah has depended, in great measure, on the medical care they receive from their doctors and other medical professionals, it has also been influenced by the evolution of public health—the organized approach we, as a society, use to care for whole populations rather than individuals.

From its early days in 1893, when nurse Lillian Wald moved to New York's Lower East Side to better understand the health challenges faced by destitute families, public health has educated the public about some of the most overwhelming impediments to health and helped to remedy them. Truly, one of public health's greatest challenges—and achievements—has been to address not only disease, but also the health disparities caused by poverty, prejudice, and other barriers.

On November 4, 1977, when former Vice President Hubert Humphrey spoke at the dedication of the national Health and Human Services building named in his honor, he reminded us all what it means to be a moral society and the important role public health plays in that endeavor. He said, "It was once said that the moral test of government is how it treats those who are in the dawn of life, the children; those who are in the twilight of life, the aged; and those in the shadows of life, the sick, the needy and the handicapped."[22]

According to the Centers for Disease Control and Prevention (CDC), we have made important strides toward this end: between 1900 and 1999, the life expectancy of people living in the United States increased by twenty-five years thanks to public health.

In Ukiah, the health of the population has depended on the quality of its private medical services, the county government's health and human services, and Ukiah's community benefit organizations—the non-profits that have continually risen to meet global problems on a local scale.

Dr. H. O. Cleland in front of Eagle Stables in 1914.

Dr. Herschel Orville Cleland

A HISTORY FROM THE CLELAND FAMILY ARCHIVES

Dr. "H. O." Cleland was born at home in 1890 in the Oak Knoll area south of Ukiah. After growing up in Ukiah, he moved to San Francisco to work and attend medical school. In 1912, he graduated from Cooper Medical College (later Stanford University Medical School) and returned to Ukiah to practice medicine for almost forty years.

In 1917, he married Francis Marguerite Thomas, daughter of W. P. Thomas, a prominent Ukiah attorney. Marguerite managed the business side of the medical practice and served as a practical nurse at the office, which was located at 203 West Standley Street, two blocks from their home at 302 West Henry Street.

At this time, many of Ukiah's streets were unpaved and schoolchildren walked or rode their horses or donkeys to school. Nurse Carolyn Brown tells of her mother riding a donkey to school and a schoolmate who used a rope bridge to ford the Russian River every morning to get to school. One-room and two-room schoolhouses dotted the landscape, so local children had to travel only a mile or two to get to school.

During the 1920s, Dr. Cleland served the community as a general practitioner in private practice; he was a skilled surgeon and a particularly keen diagnostician. In 1931, he accepted the Board of Supervisors' offer to be the superintendent of the County Hospital and Farm. As such, he was responsible for more than just medical care. He ministered to the indigent ill, including the thirty or so hospitalized patients and those convalescing at home. After being deputized, Dr. Cleland worked with the sheriff's department, allowing petty criminals and public inebriates to work off their sentences at the County Farm. Dr. Cleland also immunized school children, oversaw the indigents who lived on the farm premises, and managed the business side of the hospital and farm. Dr. Cleland was on call twenty-four hours a day, seven days a week, and in 1931, he was paid an annual salary of $1,800 for his services (equivalent to about $28,000 in 2016).

According to his family, Dr. Cleland became the target of political reformists, prompting a grand jury investigation into his work at the County Hospital. He was indicted in October 1941. The grand jury charged Dr. Cleland with letting prisoners escape (when, in fact, they were leaving the grounds during the day on their work details) and inappropriately billing the county for providing medical care and delivery services to indigent pregnant women (as it turned out, Dr. Cleland provided the care at the direction of county supervisors).

After two jury trials, both resulting in acquittals, and a favorable decision by the California Supreme Court, Dr. Cleland was fully exonerated in August 1942. As his attorney and cousin, Lilburn Gibson, said, "It had been pretty well established that these actions constituted persecution instead of prosecution."

With his grand jury woes behind him, Dr. Cleland was able to get back to the business of doctoring. When asked how he successfully managed his many responsibilities, his cousin said he responded, "I was up at five o'clock in the morning and busy all day until going to sleep at ten o'clock at night."

The challenge of running a hospital and de facto welfare department was a difficult job on the best of days, and many community members criticized his work, especially toward the end of his tenure.

In 1951, Dr. Cleland retired. He then spent winters enjoying the sunshine of Southern California, and in the spring and summer he tended his pear ranch in Potter Valley. On April 29, 1961, Dr. Cleland succumbed to a heart attack while working in his backyard at 416 Walnut Street in Ukiah.

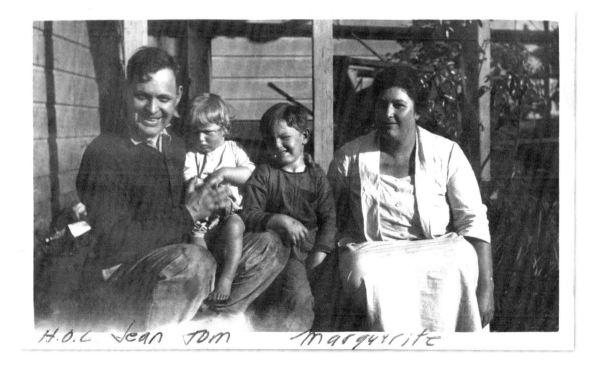

Dr. H. O. Cleland with his first wife, Marguerite, and their children Jean and Tom.

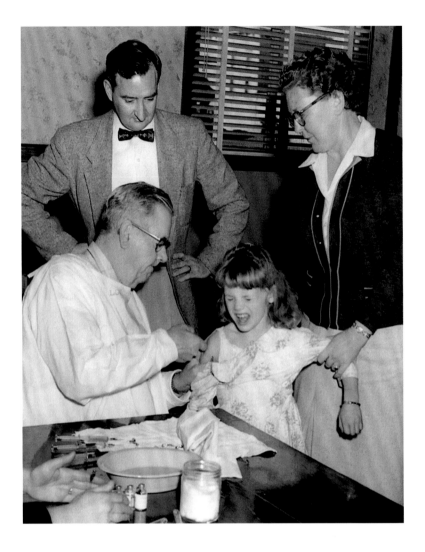

Since shots have existed, children have dreaded them. Public Health Officer Dr. Krueger and nurse Margaret Bernard administer vaccine to a young girl at Mendocino County Public Health.

In the first half of the twentieth century, the homeless and hungry of Ukiah often received assistance from volunteers in the faith community. The indigent received health care at the County Hospital and Farm from doctors such as Dr. H. O. Cleland.

Government-sponsored health care and social services were eventually divided and managed separately. Health care was split into three distinct branches: social services, public health, and mental health.

Social Services focuses on helping individuals and families improve their personal and financial self-sufficiency and protects vulnerable populations. Public health addresses issues relating to population health, such as offering preventive medicine, combating infectious and chronic diseases, and promoting healthy lifestyles and environments. Mental health concentrates on helping mentally ill people manage their conditions and provides services when mentally ill people pose a threat to themselves or others.

SOCIAL SERVICES

In the 1970s, a dedicated and skillful public administrator named Dennis Denny helped define the local role of social services by looking beyond immediate problems to their underlying causes, and he encouraged people to come together to address those causes. He worked hard to improve the lives of Ukiahans through a unique combination of innovation and common sense.

Denny worked in Social Services until his retirement in 1991 and continued his community involvement in the decades that followed.

Dennis Denny

SOCIAL SERVICES AND TREATING PEOPLE RIGHT

Dennis Denny understood what people cherished—connection with loved ones and honoring causes that spoke to their hearts—and he tapped into their desire to help one another.

As the Social Services director, Denny's top priorities were in-home services for the aged, child protective services, and combating domestic violence. However, he believed that before he could attend to those goals, he should first support his employees. High morale led to high performance, and he was dedicated to both.

In the 1970s, Denny encouraged programs in the workplace and in the community that are now commonplace but were practically unheard of back then, including what he called "adaptable" schedules. Many young women with children worked in his department, and they needed both employment and flexibility. He allowed his employees to share a single caseload and to work from home when they needed to; this simply was not done at the time, and many questioned his wisdom. He also implemented a forty-hour workweek made up of four ten-hour days so his employees could have one day a week off when doctors' offices and stores were open. Ninety percent of his employees took advantage of the four-day workweek.

"You can't believe how difficult it was; all of these concepts were very difficult to get past five supervisors, who had the right to vote whether we could do this. Oh, boy," he said, shaking his head, remembering the county supervisors who feared Social Services employees would be at home caring for their children rather than working.

Morale soared, and the Mendocino County Social Services Department was ranked among the highest in the state. "Our quality control was excellent. We got award after award after award," he said. By supporting his employees, Denny enabled them to support the clients they served, helping individuals and families improve their personal and financial self-sufficiency.

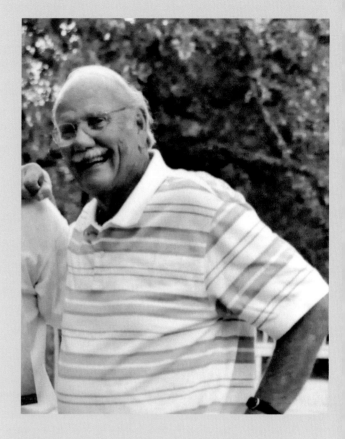

Denny was ahead of his time, supporting his employees with flexible schedules and allowing them to work from home. His decision making was ruled by compassion and a fierce dedication to his employees and those they served.

One of the reasons the department was so successful was because of its vigilance against fraud. Denny always had a talent for spotting fraud. When he was first appointed as Social Services director, he reviewed department data and noticed that the Ukiah area had an unusually high number of board and care facilities for a rural community of its size.

When he inquired as to why, he was told that, because of the state's deinstitutionalization, patients from the Mendocino State Hospital were being moved into community-based care. Privately, employees shared that Jim Jones and his People's Temple had placed disciples in strategic positions in Social Services and elsewhere, and they were funneling patients into board and care facilities managed by church members and that the funding for their care was supporting what was later identified as a cult. "Jones had

a cash cow—I mean a cash cow," Denny said.

When Denny discovered that Jones' wife, Marcy, had secured a position at the State Hospital as the out-patient placement nurse and that three high-ranking church members were working with her in Social Services to place patients into church-controlled board and care facilities, Denny reassigned those caseloads overnight—grabbing the attention of Jim Jones.

Jones requested a meeting with Denny and said he planned to bring his lawyer (the lawyer's wife was a Social Services employee). Denny met with Jones; he laid out the facts, demonstrating inappropriate use of government funds, and Jones' lawyer advised Jones to say nothing. "They just got up and walked out," Denny said. He kept a watchful eye out for further involvement from the People's Temple.

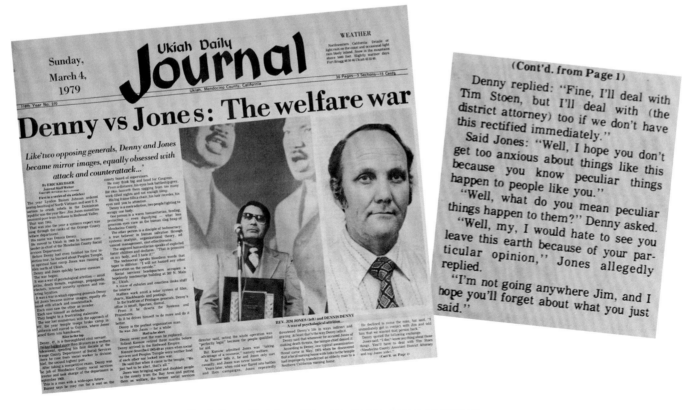

Dennis Denny did what was right, even in the face of not-so-subtle threats.

A few years later, in November 1978, after Jones had left Redwood Valley and moved to Guyana with hundreds of followers, he led more than nine hundred people to their deaths in what he called a "revolutionary suicide." Some church members drank the cyanide-laced, grape-flavored Flavor Aid voluntarily; others drank it at gunpoint. More than three hundred children were included in the murder/suicide.

While the Jim Jones situation was the most dramatic, Denny's fight against fraud was one of the hallmarks of his tenure. When the Social Services department sent fraud cases to the district attorney's office for prosecution, they never lost. Denny credits then Deputy District Attorney David Eyster's skill and dedication and the good work of his employees for their success.

As Mendocino County Social Services Director, Denny continued to advocate for populations who could not advocate for themselves. He provided county funding to support the domestic violence shelter, Project Sanctuary, and served as the chairperson of the Project Sanctuary board upon his retirement. He was also the first to contract for in-home supportive services for the elderly. This program allowed seniors who wanted to remain in their homes to do so for as long as possible; it had the added benefit of reducing the cost of nursing home care.

As director of Social Services, Denny regularly saw the long-term effects of unplanned pregnancies, so he encouraged the county to create a class on the Ukiah High School campus for young women who became pregnant that allowed them to finish their studies and graduate. Twenty of the first twenty-two students in that class finished high school. He then helped start a low-cost day care center at Mendocino College so those young mothers could continue their educations.

To help prevent unwanted pregnancies, Denny required those who applied for social services assistance to first go to family planning. While controversial, this helped reduce the financial burden on poor families who were stressed by the need to care for additional unplanned children; it also reduced the cost to Social Services to assist them.

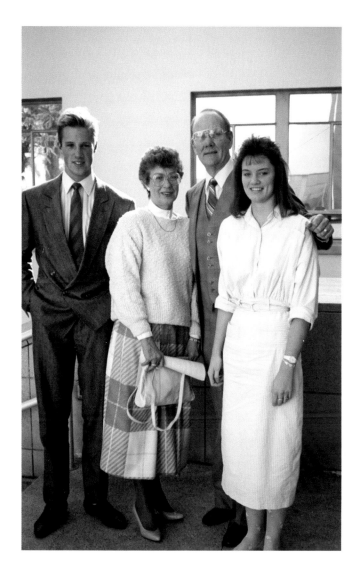

Dennis Denny pictured with his wife Patricia and their children Doug and Kristi.

By addressing some of the social determinants of health, such as greater access to education, improved economic stability, and safer environments, Denny helped people with their immediate needs and, often more importantly, provided a foundation for them to achieve long-lasting improvements in their lives. He did so in his role as Social Services director as well as through his volunteer service as a Ukiah Unified School Board member, coach for youth sports, and community leader to whom people turned when they needed help.

As a community volunteer, Denny enlisted others to make the community better. For example, when the Alex R. Thomas Plaza was created in the middle of downtown, the planners ran out of money before they had planted any trees. They approached Denny to see if he might have ideas on how the trees could be funded, and Denny recommended allowing people whose children had passed away to plant a tree in remembrance.

Denny approached local landscaper Richard Shoemaker to provide an estimate on the cost of planting big trees. He then spoke with individuals he knew who had lost children—they did not hesitate to fund the trees. A plaque with the children's names was placed on the south wall of the main park building, and just like that, the park was full of trees.

"Then we did it again," he said. The Redwood Empire Fairgrounds president wanted to plant shade trees along the main fairgrounds pathway but did not have the funds to do so. Denny and fellow community member Dede Ledford asked community members to help, and they responded in abundance.

Parnum Paving donated a large rock. Local mortuary owner Eddie Eversole provided a brass plaque and engraved the names of the donors who paid for a tree to be planted in honor of their deceased loved one. And "Memory Lane" came to life, with a hundred trees shading fairgoers for generations to come.

"This is community; we create magical moments and memories. We don't rely on others to do that for us. We here choose happiness, kindness, generosity, and empathy to all," he said.

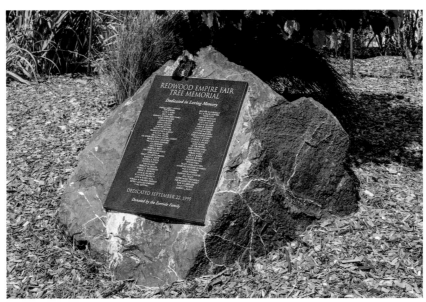

This plaque commemorates the Redwood Empire Fair Tree Memorial. More than one hundred trees were paid for by community members to commemorate their loved ones.

PUBLIC HEALTH

While Denny was helping individuals and families achieve greater personal and economic independence, the Public Health department was facing one of the biggest health challenges of modern history: the AIDS epidemic.

In the mid-1980s, patients began developing unusual illnesses such as cryptococcal meningitis and Kaposi sarcoma, baffling internists across the country until *Scientific American* published its 1986 article about the first human retro-virus: acquired immune deficiency syndrome (AIDS). Thus began a terrifying and heartbreaking period in the history of health care in Ukiah and across the nation.

Internist Dr. Marvin Trotter, who worked at Mendocino Community Hospital and in the emergency departments of General Hospital and later Ukiah Valley Medical Center, remembers the challenge of identifying some of the illnesses and the anguish of having no good treatments available to help his patients. "People would get the 'San Francisco flu' two weeks after they were exposed to the virus. Then about two years would pass before AIDS symptoms started showing up," Dr. Trotter explained. Dozens of people in Ukiah died.

Medicine changed after the AIDS epidemic. Hospitals began requiring health care workers to use more protective exposure precautions, including safety needles and surgical gloves, with all patients, not just those with communicable diseases.

In 1987, to help AIDS patients in Ukiah, Dr. Trotter joined mid-level providers Lynn Meadows and Deborah Mead as well as his wife at the time, Dr. Mary Newkirk, in establishing the Mendocino County AIDS Virus Network, later renamed the Mendocino County AIDS/Viral Hepatitis Network (MCAVHN). Mead served as the organization's executive director for thirteen years, working to stop the transmission of HIV and to care for those infected with it. Initially, MCAVHN was simply a place where AIDS patients could go for information and support. With government

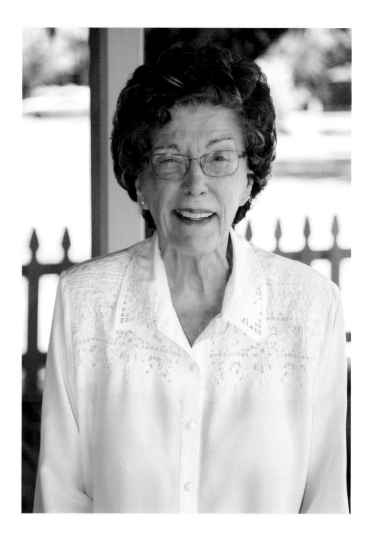

When Mendocino County AIDS Virus Network volunteers tried to start an AIDS shelter, no one would rent to them until they met local lawyer Myrna Ogelsby. Ogelsby not only rented a house to them, she also remodeled it to include two additional bedrooms and a wheelchair ramp to better meet their needs.

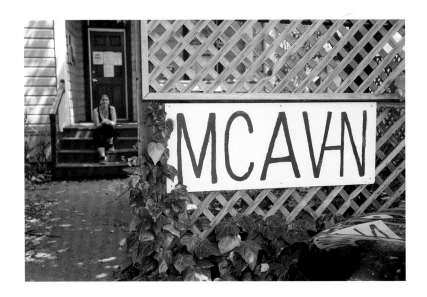

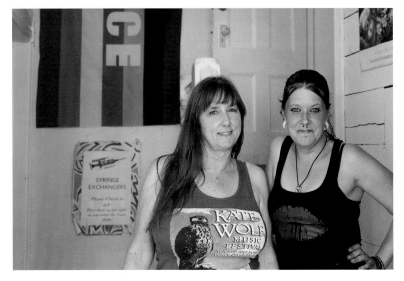

funding, however, the organization grew to provide needle exchange services, housing support, and more.

According to the 2010 Mendocino County Health Status Report, between 1982 and 2009 the county served 575 patients with HIV/AIDS. Of those individuals, 24 percent (135 people) were still living.

When federal funding for AIDS treatment ceased in the late 2000s, MCAVHN turned to the local community for support, hosting an annual fundraiser called Event of the Heart. Now, almost thirty years after its founding, MCAVHN continues to support people living with AIDS and hepatitis C. As of 2016, its executive director, Libby Guthrie, remains a strong advocate for a harm-reduction approach that embraces people with dignity and without judgment, and tries to help stabilize them physically and emotionally.

While AIDS had the full attention of those in public health, it was not the only issue requiring thoughtful and skillful administration. Fortunately for the people of Ukiah and Mendocino County, in 1991 the county hired Carol Mordhorst to oversee its Public Health department.

MCAVHN uses a harm-reduction approach, providing clients with acceptance, encouragement, and education.

Top: Employee Cynthia "Cin" Rattey assists with the MCAVHN needle exchange program.

Bottom: MCAVHN Executive Director Libby Guthrie (left) and Cin Rattey (right).

Carol Mordhorst

PUBLIC HEALTH AND COLLABORATING FOR CARE

Carol Mordhorst joined Public Health as the county was closing its hospital and health clinics but still managing all of its other responsibilities: combating infectious disease and educating the public about all manner of health threats. She was the first non-physician administrator of Public Health; since then, responsibility for Public Health has been split between a non-clinical administrator and a physician serving as a Public Health officer.

As with every other aspect of health care, public or private, county health priorities were driven in large part by funding. Upon her arrival in 1991, Mordhorst worked with local health advocates and medical providers to assess Mendocino County's greatest needs, and then sought grant funding and community support for projects that the county could not afford with its limited resources.

Mordhorst was not afraid to implement innovative or controversial programs, some of which she developed as a result of her previous public health experience in Arizona. She set up the Mendocino County Public Health Advisory Board (MCPHAB), creating a public forum to vet ideas and glean information about public health concerns and providing her with the political support she needed to implement controversial ideas such as the needle exchange program.

"We did some exciting things. We were pursuing APEX, the Assessment Protocol for Excellence in Public Health, and [MCPHAB] was part of that. [Later,] we dealt with GMOs; we dealt with the methadone clinic. You know, we tackled the Precautionary Principle. There was a lot of cutting edge stuff that was really vetted and developed at the community level, which was then taken to the board [of supervisors] and adopted," Mordhorst said.

Mordhorst helped coordinate the Rural Challenge, collecting zip code-level health data and encouraging dialogue among hundreds of participants about the particular challenges facing rural

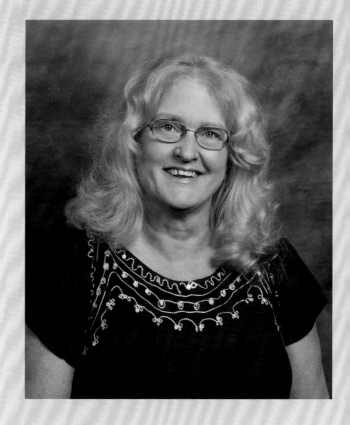

Carol Mordhorst has been working to improve public health in Ukiah since 1991 through collaboration, improved communication, technology, and innovative programs.

Northern California. Not long after, she began a publication called the Community Health Status Report (CHSR, referred to as the "cheeser"), which reviewed determinants of health in Mendocino County. Working with Ukiah Valley Medical Center, Mendocino Community Health Clinic, Consolidated Tribal Health, the Mendocino County Office of Education, and others, Public Health compared local health trends against state averages, and this collaborative effort became a key source of information for hospitals, health centers, government agencies, and non-profits in prioritizing how best to use local health care funds. The report was published every two years between 1996 and 2012. In 2014, it was supplanted by a similarly collaborative effort funded largely by the county and Ukiah Valley Medical Center: a website (www.healthy-mendocino.org) with regular updates on local, state, and national health indicators and articles relevant to population health.

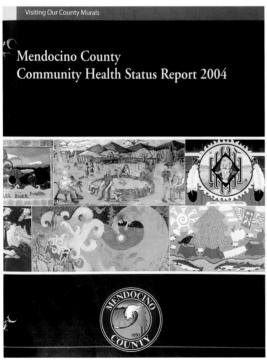

As the California state economy declined in the late 1980s and early 1990s, county funding changed, requiring creative approaches to support new programs and keep existing ones viable. Traditionally, counties had received state money and distributed it as they saw fit. In the early 1990s, California underwent "realignment," and state funding for health and human services was supplanted with dedicated revenue from sales tax and vehicle license fees. When the economy declined, people bought fewer cars and fewer goods, so the income fell short. Eventually, however, the economy recovered, and the dedicated funding stream (which was not allowed to become part of the county's general fund) allowed Social Services, Mental Health, and Public Health to invest in infrastructure, long-term planning, and new programs. In 2009, the county was able to purchase the building at 1120 South Dora Street that was once Ukiah General Hospital. This became Public Health's new home.

Mordhorst recognized that even in good times, public demand for services would outstrip county resources, so she worked with community partners to choose four priority areas, focusing limited Public Health resources on access to care, healthy lifestyles, drug and alcohol treatment, and aging.

"One of the more significant issues was access to care," Mordhorst said. She explained that, as a fee-for-service county, poor families could seek care from any doctor who accepted Medi-Cal's public insurance, but this was problematic for two reasons: first, many doctors opted not to see patients covered by Medi-Cal because of its low reimbursement, and second, many families did not qualify for Medi-Cal, either because they made slightly too much money (and so went without insurance) or because they were undocumented. For Mordhorst and others, this was especially troubling for poor children in Mendocino County.

This led Mordhorst to work with Cathy Frey at the Alliance for Rural Community Health (a consortium of Federally Qualified Health Centers), Anne Molgaard at First 5 Mendocino (a state-funded non-profit designed to support the healthy development of children from birth to age five), and other local child and health care advocates to create Healthy Kids Mendocino, with the goal of providing health insurance for all children living in Mendocino County. Healthy Kids Mendocino provided coverage for children in Ukiah and throughout the county until it was no longer needed because of the Affordable Care Act in 2010 and other state and federal health insurance initiatives. In 2016, a program called Carrots still existed for any Mendocino County child who does not qualify for other public health insurance programs.

Another important way the county improved access to care was through its collaborative emergency medical service (EMS), working with medical transport companies and hospital emergency departments to make sure local people could get timely emergency care. Mordhorst brokered an agreement with Sonoma County to create a joint EMS region, upgrading Mendocino County's basic life support (BLS) to advanced cardiac life support (ACLS). This meant emergency personnel received additional training so they could do more than simply pick up a patient and rush them to a hospital (BLS training only allows for basic resuscitation and rescue). ACLS training enabled emergency medical technicians and paramedics to use life-saving techniques and medications for patients whose conditions could prove fatal before an ambulance could get them safely to the hospital.

Whether providing emergency transport or managing other health challenges, Public Health was often called upon to respond. While AIDS, tuberculosis, and other diseases continued to endanger patients in Ukiah, new threats emerged—nationwide and worldwide—such as bio-terrorism and pandemic flu. And after the tragic events of September 11, 2001, when terrorists attacked the United States, significant funding was made available to prepare for and hopefully prevent disasters. "There was all this stuff about anthrax; for example, if there was pandemic flu, how were we going to deploy our staff, or how were we going to deploy that medication—we might have to vaccinate the entire population in forty-eight hours," Mordhorst said.

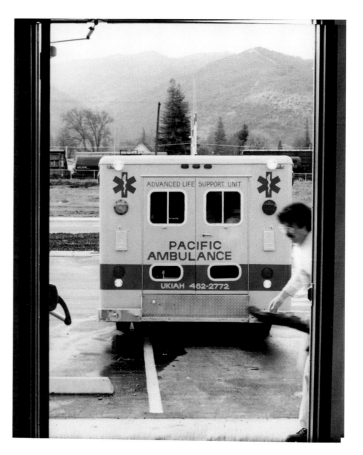

Carol Mordhorst encouraged the creation of a collaborative emergency medical service in Mendocino County.

Tabletop simulations and full-blown disaster drills included countywide emergency medical responders as well as law enforcement, teaching local organizations how best to communicate and collaborate during a crisis. Hospital personnel learned to use the same incident command system that government and law enforcement personnel used during an emergency, and trailers stocked with disaster supplies (cots, tents, bandages, and more) were placed throughout the county.

Whether it was disaster drills, EMS contracts, or finding ways to fund health insurance for children, Mordhorst believed in collaborating. She even encouraged the county to bring the three health branches under a single agency, the Health and Human Services Agency, to improve quality through better communication and streamlined goals. Unfortunately, the integration was not a smooth process, and after fifteen years with the county, Mordhorst decided to resign and begin her own consulting firm.

Mordhorst continued to work in the health industry in Ukiah, consulting with Partnership HealthPlan of California to bring Medi-Cal managed care to Mendocino County; volunteering on the board of Manzanita Services, a non-profit community benefit organization assisting those with mental health challenges; and administering Partnership HealthPlan for the Alliance for Rural Community Health (ARCH). She continues in these roles in 2016, as this book goes to press.

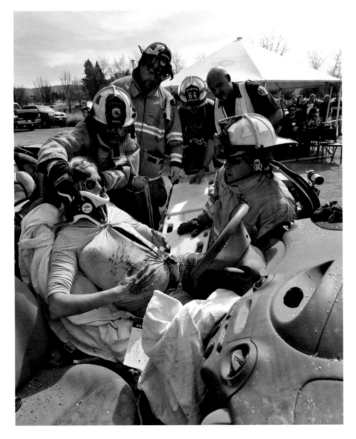

Multi-agency disaster drills began with encouragement from Carol Mordhorst, and they continue today. Pictured, emergency first responders practice while hospital nurses and others watch and learn.

The future of public health will likely follow the current trend of identifying the social determinants of health and working to reduce inequities as well as creating healthier environments through education and the funding of new and innovative projects.

Some initiatives gaining popularity nationwide include detailed food labeling so people know what they are consuming, including whether foods are genetically modified; community gardens; a soda tax to combat obesity; and city planning that includes paths for cyclists and pedestrians to decrease the need for automobile travel.

Ukiah has already adopted some of these through the work of organizations such as North Coast Opportunities, a non-profit community-building organization with programs such as Walk and Bike Mendocino (which supports efforts to make it easier and safer to walk and bike, rather than drive) and the Gardens Project (which supports neighborhood gardens).

MENTAL HEALTH

While Ukiah's public health history has much to be proud of, one area of its services has consistently struggled: mental health. In the nineteenth and early twentieth centuries, the mentally ill were commonly institutionalized, and Ukiah was home to a state mental hospital housing thousands of inpatients from 1893 to 1972. Today, failure to adequately serve its mentally ill population, while not unique to the region, has often led to disappointment—and for those with mentally ill loved ones, even heartbreak. While certain individuals shine brightly because of their valiant efforts on behalf of this population, Ukiah still works to knit together the agencies and limited resources necessary to care for those with ongoing mental health challenges.

Treating the mentally ill is complex from scientific, social, and financial standpoints. In his book *Madness in Civilization: A Cultural History of Insanity, from the Bible to Freud, from the Madhouse to Modern Medicine*, author Andrew Scull argues that mental illness has not been properly treated because, in large part, it has been (and remains) poorly understood.

Even today, there are few definitive tests to ascertain precisely what type of mental illness afflicts someone, and what, if any,

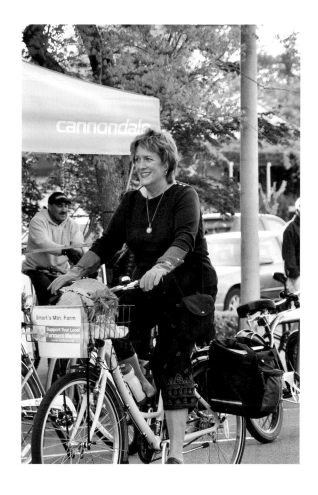

Former Ukiah Unified School Board member Peggy Smart participated in the Walk-Bike Mendocino Fashion Show in 2011, demonstrating that people could ride their bicycles in work clothes.

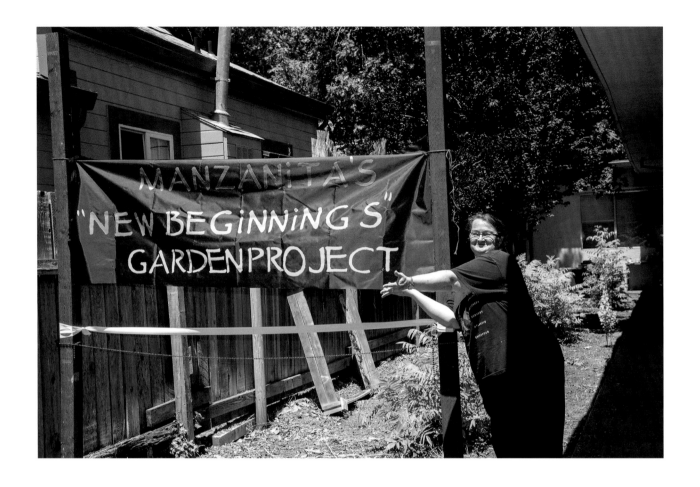

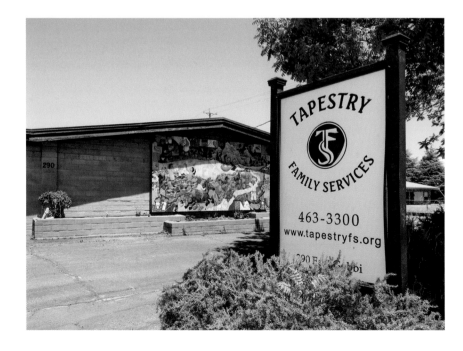

Top: Holly Smith has been a client/volunteer with Manzanita Services since its inception in 2008. Manzanita uses a peer support model to help clients gain the skills they need to overcome trauma and manage mental illness to live productive lives.

Right: Since 2001, Tapestry Family Services has served as a foster family agency and a children's mental health treatment center.

treatments might be effective. In an interview on *Consider This* on National Public Radio in August 2015, Scull explained that the earliest medications used to treat mental illness were discovered accidentally. In the 1950s, doctors noted that Thorazine had a calming effect on patients—researchers were not attempting to identify this outcome with the drug. Accidental discovery helps explain the lack of understanding about *why* a drug works. Even with the anti-depressants used to treat millions of Americans today, Scull suggests that the idea of "balancing brain chemistry" is an assumption with little scientific proof. Maybe serotonin reuptake inhibitors help rebalance the brain's chemistry; maybe they do not, he suggests. They do seem to help the symptoms of depression, and for many, that is enough. However, the side effects of those and many psychotropic medications tend to send patients in search of other options; people would like to heal, not swap one problem for another.

In addition to not truly understanding the origins and causes of mental illness, the social stigma around mental illness has often prevented people from dedicating resources to funding research and treatment.

Ukiah has struggled to serve the mentally ill since the Mendocino State Hospital closed in 1972, even though non-profit organizations such as the Mendocino Chapter of the National Alliance on Mental Illness, Manzanita Services, Redwood Community Services, and Tapestry Family Services have joined county mental health, law enforcement, and medical facilities to care for mentally ill people in the area. After the mental hospital closed, many patients were unable to integrate into the community while receiving outpatient psychiatric care.

The first director of the Mendocino County Mental Health Department was Dr. Dick Drury, who had also worked at Mendocino State Hospital. According to those who worked with him, Dr. Drury was a conscientious psychiatrist whose patient assessments were impressively thorough.

Dr. Drury preferred the clinical over the administrative side of mental health, so he eventually became the medical director and Robert Charles Egnew took over as the mental health director. During these years, mental health care in Ukiah took a positive turn. The state approved funding for the Community Support System Project, a project that encouraged county mental health

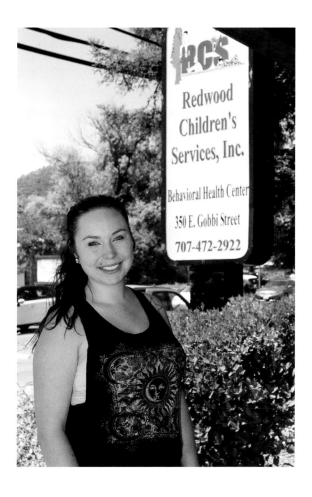

Redwood Community Services began as a foster family agency in 1995, then expanded to meet the needs of youth like Tesla Talbot (pictured above). With the help of RCS, Talbot overcame a traumatic childhood to become an RCS employee.

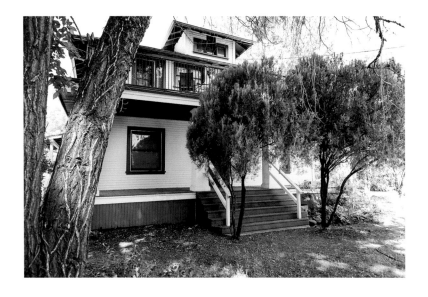

Between 1981–1989, the Bonita House in Ukiah allowed severely mentally ill people to live in a safe environment while receiving treatment.

"The Bonita House took seriously mentally ill individuals out of higher levels of care like hospitals and IMDS [institutes for mental disease] and allowed them to participate in a shared living program, where they received treatment from para-professional and professional staff. The program was successful and lasted until the funding for mental health services in the county began to decline."

–Susan Era, retired Social Services director.

departments to engage consumers in creating self-help groups and activities, and supported those groups with professional case managers who specialized in addressing the specific needs of diverse mentally ill populations, including Latinos and the elderly.[23]

Around this same time, Egnew also contracted with a non-profit organization from the Bay Area to open the Bonita House, a seven-bed licensed residential treatment facility in Ukiah for adults with persistent mental illness.

"The Bonita House took seriously mentally ill individuals out of higher levels of care like hospitals and IMDs [institutes for mental disease] and allowed them to participate in a shared living program, where they received treatment from para-professional and professional staff. The program was successful and lasted until the funding for mental health services in the county began to decline," said Susan Era, retired Social Services director. The Bonita House remained open from 1981 to 1989.

The 1980s also saw the birth of the Mendocino County chapter of the National Alliance on Mental Illness (NAMI), which had the goal of supporting, educating, and advocating for the patients, their families, and their community. When state mental health funding declined, "what became obvious was a gaping hole in treatment and housing options for those with mental illness or dementia," Era explained.

Through the 1990s, county health professionals worked with local health organizations and non-profits to care for the mentally ill, who often bounced from the hospital emergency department to the Federally Qualified Health Center, and sometimes to the jail. This is where they would meet Dr. Douglas Rosoff, the county's psychiatrist, whose personal mission was to alleviate suffering for the mentally ill.

Dr. Douglas Rosoff

A TRUE BELIEVER IN COMMUNITY HEALTH

Doug Rosoff received his bachelor's degree at Stanford University and attended medical school at the Kansas City School of Osteopathic Medicine. He completed his psychiatric residency at Westchester Medical Center in New York and UC Davis, and initially came to Ukiah to work for the county on a short-term assignment: serving the underserved to repay part of his educational debt. After fulfilling his responsibilities in Mendocino County, he left to care for underserved populations in Texas and Alaska, and when his school debt was repaid, he returned to Ukiah to take a permanent position under his mentor, Dr. Dick Drury.

Dr. Drury cared for most of the county's inpatients (patients hospitalized because of their mental illness), and Dr. Rosoff cared for most of the outpatients; the two doctors shared responsibility for mentally ill patients in the jail. Eventually, Dr. Drury left the county, and Dr. Rosoff became the medical director for County Mental Health.

Dr. Rosoff's widow, Catherine, said, "Doug was a true believer in community health and a true believer in alleviating suffering." She described the way Dr. Rosoff would treat all patients with the utmost respect, even those who were severely disturbed and behaved in completely irrational or unpleasant ways. "He would just stay calm and collect information about the solid things that mattered. Nothing was too basic for him to find out." At the same time, she explained, he set a lot of limits. She recalled one story of Dr. Rosoff telling a patient, "This is not a Chinese restaurant, buddy. You don't get to pick and choose your medications."

According to licensed clinical social worker Noel O'Neill, the psychiatrist's colleague of fifteen years, "Dr. Rosoff was an incredible forensic psychiatrist. He really had a passion for going into the jail and doing the evaluations for these people [to determine if they were competent to stand trial], and he could tell if someone was faking it versus truly psychotic."

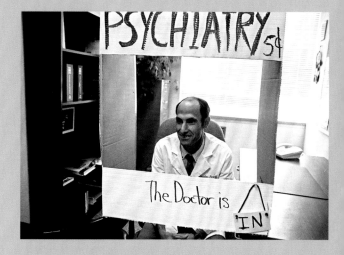

County psychiatrist Dr. Doug Rosoff is remembered for treating all patients with respect and working continuously to see that those in the jail received the treatment they needed.

Sheriff Tom Allman said he did not know Dr. Rosoff until Allman became sheriff in 2006. "When I became sheriff, I started getting notes from families that said things like, 'Please tell Dr. Rosoff how much we appreciate him allowing our son to dry out from his psychiatric medicine, and then finding out what worked for him and what didn't, and getting him back on track.'"

Dr. Rosoff spent half of his professional hours and many more personal hours working with mentally ill inmates at the county jail. When he was not at the jail, he treated patients in his office. O'Neill said Dr. Rosoff also loved to teach and gave many lectures, especially to local emergency room physicians, because of the frequency with which they encountered mentally ill patients. "He had such a passion for serving. Doug was on 24/7," O'Neill said.

In 2011, Dr. Rosoff left the county's employ and began working for the local Veteran's Administration; he was there only a short time before a bicycle accident on August 24, 2012, led to his untimely death at age fifty-six.

To honor Dr. Rosoff's service and his memory, Ukiah Valley Medical Center plans to name one of the rooms in its new emergency department after him.

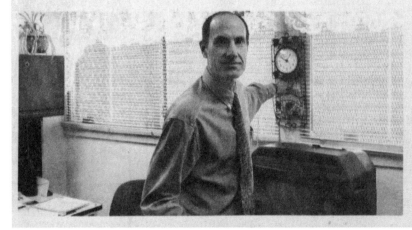

Sheriff's Office partners with the Mental Health Department

By GLENDA ANDERSON
The Daily Journal

Six months after the county Mental Health Department took over mental health services at the jail, things reportedly are going well.

"I'm just delighted with the partnership between the Sheriff's Office and Mental Health with respect to treatment in the jail," Sheriff Tony Craver said last week.

He said it only makes sense that mental health services at the jail and the county clinic be the same, for more fluid and effective treatment.

Jail mental health services had, since 1990, been provided by the California Forensic Medical Group.

CFMG continues to handle medical

See JAIL, Page 14

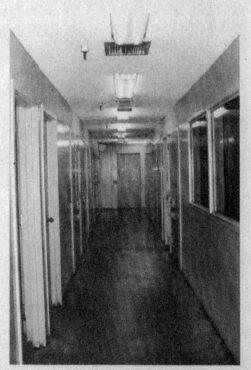

(Above) The corridor in the men's section of the jail off the sally port where incoming arrestees are brought for booking and observation. (Left) Doug Rosoff takes a visitation request slip from the in-box in the medical office at the jail.

Dr. Doug Rosoff began spending significant time, both on the clock and off, treating patients in the Mendocino County jail in 2002.

In 2004, Proposition 63, the Mental Health Services Act (MHSA), passed, providing "increased funding, personnel and other resources to support county mental health programs and monitor progress toward statewide goals for children, transition age youth, adults, older adults and families. The Act addresses a broad continuum of prevention, early intervention and service needs and the necessary infrastructure, technology and training elements that will effectively support this system," according to the Department of Mental Health website.[24] In response, Mendocino County developed community-based plans with input from consumers, family members, professionals, and collaborating partners.

O'Neill said, "Probably the biggest change that Proposition 63 made in community mental health was that it transformed that service from a medical service to a recovery model service. A recovery model uses persons who have either recovered from symptoms of mental illness or who are recovering and have learned how to manage their symptoms to help their peers. They can be so effective in helping other people. It's not an either/or—you need the professional side. You need the Doug Rosoffs of the world; you have to have that. But there's a recognition that peer-to-peer service is also really critical."

So while mental health professionals continued to treat patients, MSHA funds allowed the county to support peer-to-peer services such as Ukiah's Manzanita Services, a non-profit organization dedicated to serving those living with mental health challenges.

As the California economy struggled, the Mendocino County Mental Health department operated further into the red. Leadership of the department turned over several times, making matters worse. County health leaders worked with the board of supervisors to devise three major

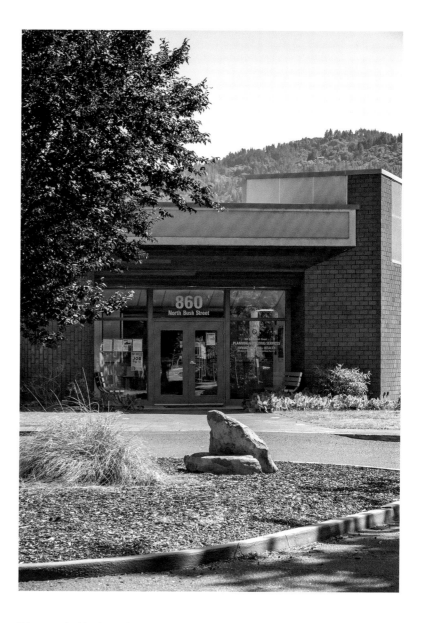

This county building housed the locked mental health facility. The abbreviation for the Public Health Facility was the "PFH Unit" (pronounced "puff unit").

PARTNERSHIP

HEALTHPLAN
of CALIFORNIA

Partnership HealthPlan of California has been praised for its administration of mild to moderate mental health care benefits for those with Medi-Cal coverage.

strategies to improve the financial picture: 1. To provide in-county treatment for mental health patients currently sent out of county for higher levels of care; 2. To maximize the use of realignment dollars for local mental health services; and 3. To bill properly for services rendered by the Mental Health department.

But because of inadequate funding and inconsistent leadership, little progress was made.

When the Affordable Care Act passed in 2010, the State of California expanded Medi-Cal benefits to include treatment of mild to moderate mental illness. Treatment for severe mental illness continued to be funded under the 1915(b) waiver (which defines complicated state funding options for some mental health services) and provided by county mental health services. Among other things, 1915(b) waivers allow counties to act as enrollment brokers to help people pick a managed care plan, as well as allowing counties to act as "choice counselors," according to the Medicaid.gov website.[25]

Partnership HealthPlan of California, which administers Medi-Cal benefits for fourteen Northern California counties including Mendocino, indicated that in 2015, Mendocino County's care of the mild to moderate mental health population was among the best in the state. This is due, in large part, to the mental health care provided through community clinics such as Hillside Health Center (part of Mendocino Community Health Clinic), the Federally Qualified Health Center in Ukiah that provides behavioral health services as well as medical and dental services, regardless of people's ability to pay.

As Partnership took over administration of mild to moderate mental health care benefits for those with Medi-Cal coverage, the county outsourced administration of care for severely mentally ill adults to the Ortner Management Group and severely mentally ill children to Redwood Quality Services. While the hospital has shared its appreciation for Ortner's responsiveness in taking mentally ill patients out of the emergency department and into a more appropriate care venue, the jury is out as to whether this outsourcing will remain the solution of choice. Ortner ceased to provide mental health services in the county as of July 2016.

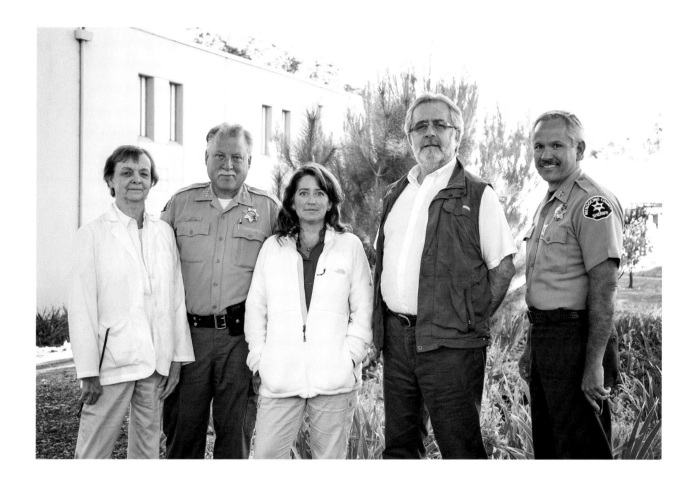

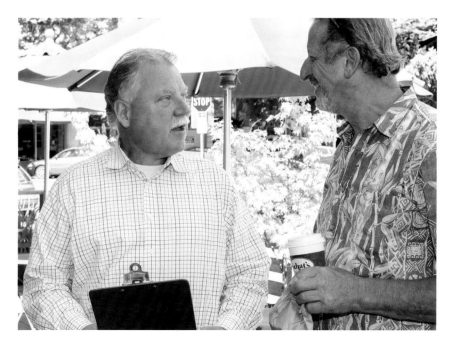

Top: Without adequate health care resources, those with mental illness often end up in the criminal justice system. Left to right: Claire Teske, RN, Medical Manager, Sheriff Tom Allman, Teresa Brassfield, RN, Behavioral Court Case Manager, Robert Hurley, RN, Mental Health Nurse, and Captain Tim Pearce, Jail Commander.

Left: Sheriff Tom Allman has worked for years to increase health care services for mentally ill people in Mendocino County. In 2016, mental health services remain under-funded. Pictured, Sheriff Tom Allman asks community member Ed Keller to sign a 2016 ballot initiative for a sales tax increase to raise money to provide additional mental health facilities in Mendocino County.

MENDOCINO COUNTY HEALTH AND HUMAN SERVICES AND POPULATION HEALTH

Stacey Cryer, director of the Health and Human Services Agency (HHSA) from 2012 to 2016, consistently lobbied for additional funding for county health services, but with little success. Cryer worked to shift Public Health priorities from direct services to population-based health focused on four goals: creating safe places for people to be physically active, ensuring access to healthy food, promoting positive role models and healthy lifestyles, and reducing violence and the fear of violence. While these are lofty goals, Cryer was confident that if government services collaborated with local health providers, community organizations, educational leaders, and law enforcement, the goals would be achievable.

The local collaboration that began after the passing of the Affordable Care Act was unprecedented. Ukiah Valley Medical Center president Gwen Matthews called it a "seismic shift." Now health care organizations that used to compete for patients had a financial model that supported coordination and collaboration, allowing them to work together for the good of the patient regardless of the setting.

With the Affordable Care Act of 2010, Congress passed the most comprehensive health care legislation in fifty years. By 2015, almost ten million Americans had signed up for health insurance through the ACA health care exchanges. During this same time, managed Medi-Cal, administered by Partnership HealthPlan of California, arrived in Mendocino County, and for the first time in decades (maybe ever), public health care funding pivoted away from episodic care toward prevention—paying medical providers to keep people healthy rather than paying them only for each patient visit.

This prospective payment system (PPS) paid health centers and hospitals a set amount per enrolled patient per month, placing the responsibility on providers to cover the cost of care and to keep patients healthy. Instead of being paid fees for providing services, the focus could now shift to coordinating and integrating care and promoting health and well-being. Clearly, medical providers and institutions saw the benefits to patients and themselves to focus on prevention and medical management rather than on crisis-based care.

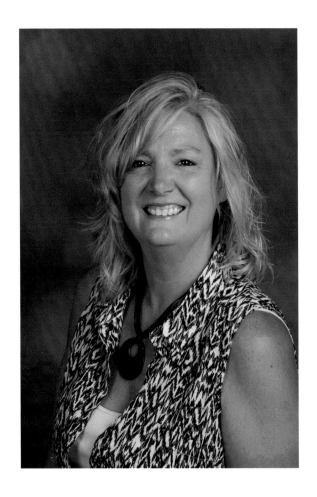

Above: Stacey Cryer served as the director of Mendocino County Health and Human Services as the county blended Public Health, Mental Health, and Social Services into one agency.

Opposite: Judith Harwood facilities a meeting to help Health and Human Services identify gaps and overlaps in health care and collaborate with community organizations to meet the needs of local people. Participants included Redwood Children's Services Executive Director Camille Schrader, HHSA employee MaryLou Leonard, HHSA Director Stacey Cryer, ARCH Executive Director Cathy Frey, local health advocate Susan Baird Kanaan, MSW, and Cancer Resources Center of Mendocino County Executive Director Sara O'Donnell, among others.

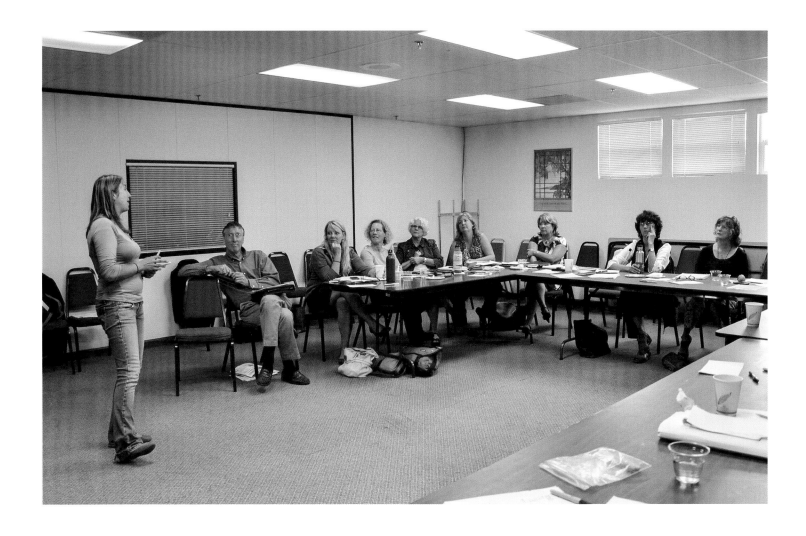

Being a "community of solution," Mendocino County has joined communities across the nation in which health, government, and community organizations work together to improve the quality of life for local residents.

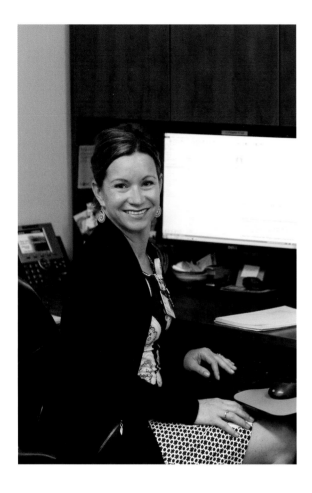

Ukiah Valley Medical Center employee Sandy O'Ferrall works with community organizations to address population health issues.

In 2013, Ukiah author and health advocate Susan Baird Kanaan, MSW, wrote an article lauding the collaboration of twenty community partners in providing "regularly updated public data on local health and its determinants from fifteen state and federal sources, along with monitoring and comparison tools and a national database of promising community health practices" through healthymendocino.org.[26] Being a "community of solution," Mendocino County has joined communities across the nation in which health, government, and community organizations work together to improve the quality of life for local residents.

This has paved the way for Mendocino County HHSA, Ukiah Valley Medical Center, Mendocino Community Health Clinic, Consolidated Tribal Health Project, and North Coast Opportunities to work together on a regional needs assessment and to communicate about shared patients and clients with the goal of helping people stay healthier (they plan to include even more organizations in the next needs assessment in 2018).

As local organizations communicated more effectively, still more opportunities for collaboration came to light. UVMC was able to provide a safe place for homeless patients discharged from the hospital by supporting the Ford Street Project's Unity Village, a place where clean and sober individuals and families can qualify for short-term housing. UVMC funded four respite beds at Unity Village, which was wonderful for patients and had the added benefit of providing Ford Street with more funding.

Sandy O'Ferrall, UVMC's representative on the HHSA community advisory board, said she has been impressed by the way organizations are connecting for the good of patients. She told the story of a heroin addict who was continually readmitted to the hospital until UVMC and the Ukiah Community Center began working together on the patient's behalf. Through intensive case management, the patient was able to achieve some stability in his life, keeping him out of the hospital and on the road to recovery.

"We have incredible resources for people in Ukiah," O'Ferrall said. She added that she enjoys being the point person for the collaborative needs assessment process and is encouraged by what she believes are building blocks for long-term collaboration.

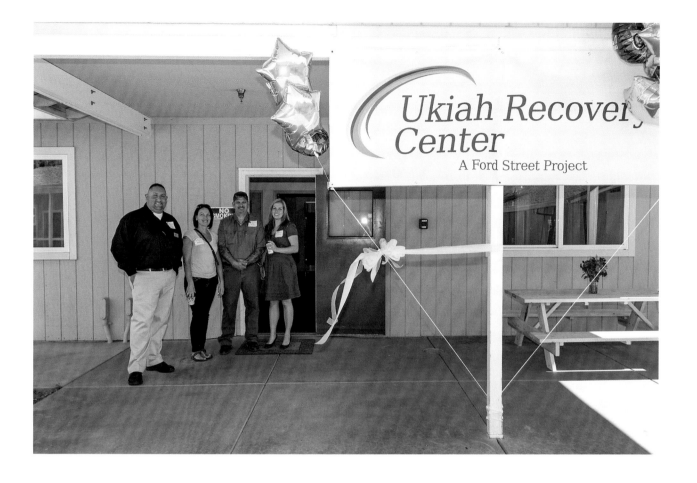

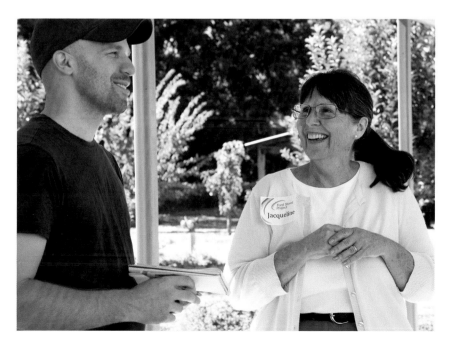

Top: Ukiah Recovery Center, a service of the Ford Street Project, provides an inpatient drug and alcohol rehabilitation center where clients can overcome addictions. Pictured, employees celebrate during the rehabilitation center's grand opening on October 16, 2015.

Left: Ford Street Project Executive Director Jacque Williams talks with *Ukiah Daily Journal* reporter Adam Randall during the Ukiah Recovery Center grand opening.

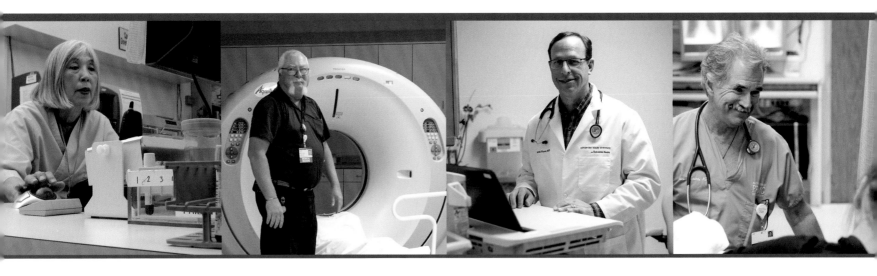

Over time, the focus of medicine has shifted from infectious diseases to chronic diseases, then to the prevention of diseases based on a broader understanding of what makes individuals and communities healthy.

The Future of Health Care

Historians often look to the past to predict the future, as history has proven to be an excellent teacher. For health care, history may indeed hold the keys to the future as we come full circle—returning attention to patients' personal health and well-being.

At the turn of the twentieth century, general practitioners treated all of their patients' health problems. GPs typically knew their patients' medical history as well as their social and emotional stressors and would use all of this information to provide integrated, whole-person care with the limited health expertise available at the time.

As specialization increased, patients benefited from medical breakthroughs but suffered from a fragmented system in which individuals received care from several practitioners who were not always aware of all the factors influencing a patient's health. During this same period, public health focused on combating infectious disease but paid relatively little attention to the upstream causes of why some populations were healthier than others.

Today, medical care is evolving to incorporate the benefits of whole-person care (physical, social, emotional, and spiritual) with the highly specialized medical knowledge and technology now available. Over time, the focus of medicine has shifted from infectious diseases to chronic diseases, then to the prevention of diseases based on a broader understanding of what makes individuals and communities healthy. Community health is using the social determinants of health to move away from direct services and, instead, to change social and political structures with the goal of decreasing health disparities. Social determinants of health include medical care, education, economic stability, the physical and built environments, and a person's social and community context. In this age of information, best practices from all over the world can be quickly shared and integrated into modern medicine.

Opposite Left: Lab technician Kimi Oliveira uses the computer to review data.

Opposite Center Left: Medical Imaging technician Mike Falge prepares to scan a patient using the CT scanner.

Opposite Center Right: Dr. David Ploss uses the computer to update patient charts. Paper charts are no longer used.

Opposite Right: Emergency Room physician Dr. Charlie Evans uses an ultrasound machine to evaluate a patient's arm injury.

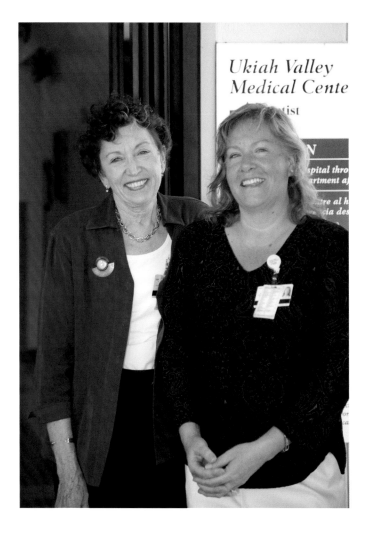

Diabetes Educators Brenda Hoek, RN, and Linda Ayotte, RD, CDE, work with patients to help them develop healthier habits.

While there is much cause for optimism, some health problems remain stubbornly intractable. At the same time that medical breakthroughs have created new and exciting cancer-fighting drugs and the mapping of the human genome suggests we may be able to prevent or reverse the effects of inherited disorders, the problems caused by issues as basic as physical inactivity and poor nutrition have led to an obesity epidemic in which a third of all American adults are at higher risk for type 2 diabetes, heart disease, and some forms of cancer as compared to their normal-weight counterparts.[27] Sadly, unprecedented numbers of children also suffer from obesity, including 43 percent of Mendocino County youth.[28] It is a powerful statement that this is the first generation predicted to have a shorter life expectancy than the one before, largely due to obesity and diabetes.[29]

Hospital president Gwen Matthews said, "We are living in an amazing time. We now know that genetic markers, once thought to determine the course of health and illness, can be suppressed by healthy lifestyle practices. We can turn off disease markers to live longer, healthier lives if we eat well, exercise, and reduce stress and trauma in our lives."

While technology cannot supplant education and the collective willpower to make healthy lifestyle choices, it has led to breakthroughs such as the human papilloma virus vaccine, robotic surgery, the first face transplant, stem cell research, nanotechnology, and a substantial expansion of health care information technology. Scientists have also gone toe-to-toe with bacteria in an effort to keep up with bacteria's ability to evolve and survive against constantly changing antibiotics. Drug-resistant bacteria have wreaked havoc in many hospitals, where modern doctors feel much like the doctors of old—clearly understanding the problem but unable to do much about it.

At Ukiah Valley Medical Center, local physicians and staff connected with infectious disease specialist Dr. Javeed Siddiqui in Roseville, California and collaborated to alter the course of micro-organisms that were resistant to antibiotics, re-sensitizing them to treatment through judicious use and good stewardship of antibiotics.

With the explosion of computer technology and its ever-expanding ability to store and retrieve more data more quickly, access to care in the twenty-first century has become intertwined with the age of information, and in some ways access to information has become synonymous with access to care.

Since the turn of the twenty-first century, UVMC has invested heavily in computerized information systems, including Cerner's electronic medical records and the Picture Archiving and Communication System for digital transmission of all imaging. This has allowed physicians to share patient information with colleagues instantaneously and to compare their patients' old data with new data without having to wait for hours (or days) while hospital staff search for archived test results.

The digitalization of radiology and pathology has allowed experts from major teaching hospitals and other institutions to assist on tough cases in remote, rural locations, saving lives in the process.

"Right now, right here in town, when pathologists have a question, they send information to St. Helena Hospital or down to Los Angeles over the Internet for instantaneous feedback," said recently retired pathologist Dr. Herschel Gordon. "I used to send information to Clarient, a reference lab owned by GE [General Electric], and would get second opinions from experts from all over." Clarient served as a clearinghouse, finding the best-qualified pathologist for the specific type of tissue to be analyzed. Especially with aggressive forms of cancer and other diseases that spread rapidly, the sooner the doctors understand the pathology of a specimen, the more quickly they can prescribe the proper treatment to give patients the best chance of a full recovery.

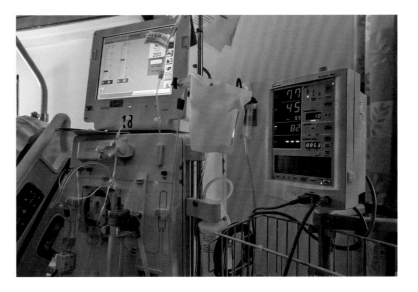

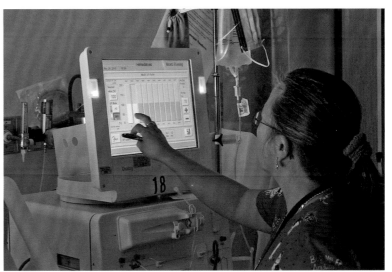

Top: Health care professionals use computers to monitor patients' conditions. Automatic alarms sound if a patient's condition deteriorates.

Bottom: In 2016, Ukiah Valley Medical Center contracted with Dialysis Clinic, Inc. to provide hemodialysis to patients. Pictured: Nurse Avelina Pottinger reviews a patient's data.

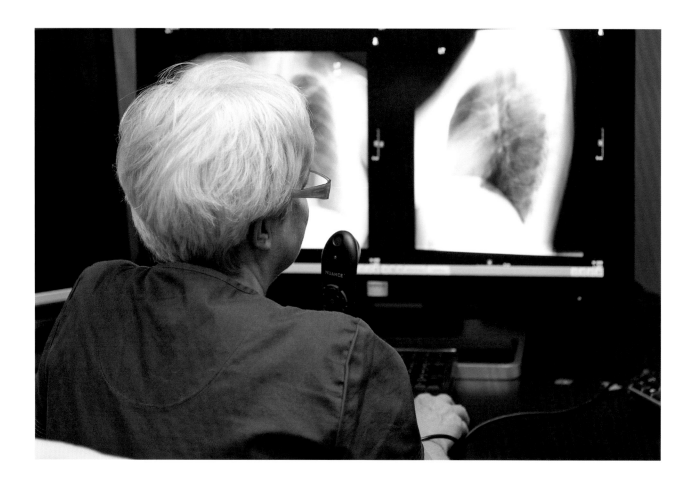

Top: Radiologist Dr. Laura Winkle dictates her report while reviewing digital images.

Right: Physician Assistant Lisa Gamble dictates patient data into the electronic medical record.

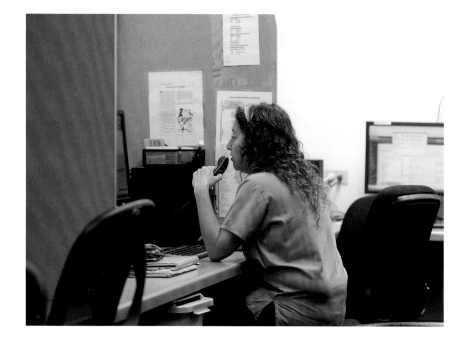

The same technology applies to computerized axial tomography (CAT) scans, positron emission tomography (PET) scans, and digital X-rays. "We can communicate with people anywhere in the world to get a second opinion without waiting for the mailman to deliver the data," Dr. Gordon explained.

Another way for rural communities such as Ukiah to benefit from specialists and sub-specialists who cannot support themselves without a major population base is through telemedicine. For a time, UVMC collaborated with critical care specialist Dr. James Gude in Santa Rosa to care for patients using a robot to transmit information. In the Ukiah Valley Medical Center emergency department and intensive care unit, a patient with symptoms indicating a serious problem could be "seen" by Dr. Gude. A stethoscope was connected to the robot so Dr. Gude could hear a heartbeat as though he were in the room with the patient. High-resolution images were transmitted through a video camera in the robot's "face" so Dr. Gude could see and talk to the patient, conversing in real time. Blended with the ability to share lab and imaging results in moments via the Internet, Dr. Gude had everything he needed to diagnose a patient's condition and recommend a course of action. Because Dr. Gude was rarely seen without his signature bow tie, the folks at UVMC put a bow tie on the robot, too.

Even aside from the ability to involve physicians from outside Ukiah, the technology of electronic medical records has improved care by making information available with the push of a button, thereby reducing errors, including the misinterpretation of handwritten doctors' orders.

Lynn Chevalier, executive assistant to several hospital presidents, compared the handwriting of one of her favorite physicians to that of a "disabled, left-handed chicken." Hospital employees from other departments would sometimes come to Administration to ask Chevalier or medical staff director Betty Rae Jose if they could confidently interpret what a doctor had written, because orders could not be carried out until they were sure.

Electronic medical records have also improved patient safety by flagging possible medication errors or dangerous combinations of medications prescribed by multiple physicians who are unaware of each other's prescriptions. Access to more information has quickly translated into better care for patients.

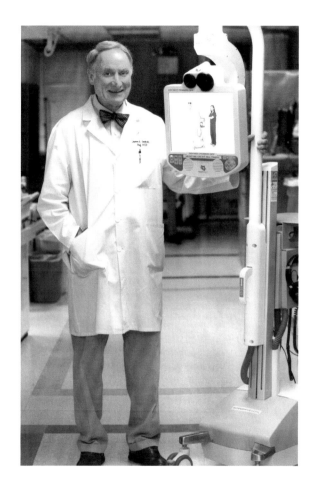

Critical care specialist Dr. James Gude worked remotely to assist Ukiah Valley Medical Center patients via a robot.

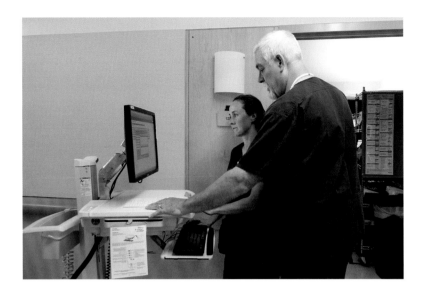

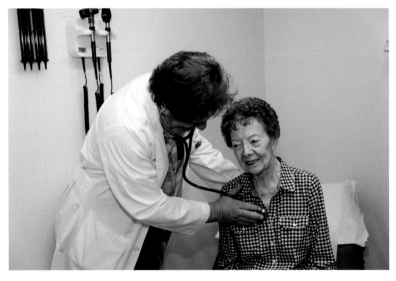

Gains in efficiency, though, have sometimes been offset by imperfect software. Doctors have complained about the difficulty of entering non-standard or narrative information. They say check boxes and templates are not adequate replacements for a physician's free-flowing summary of a patient's condition—a summary they could read and absorb in moments. However, as software improves, these complaints dwindle. Even with its shortcomings, electronic medical records have improved care coordination and patient safety.

While technology continued to provide ever-increasing access to information, some people in Ukiah did not have access to those benefits because they could not get in to see a doctor due to a shortage of physicians in the area. To address this problem, the hospital supported community efforts to bring more primary care physicians to the community. However, primary care physicians were in short supply nationwide and were not choosing to practice in rural areas. This led Gwen Matthews and Chief of Staff Dr. Charlie Evans to actively pursue creating a family medicine residency program, in hopes of retaining some of the physicians they train.

Top: Nurses Iva Jo Otto, RN, and Ron Pike, RN, confer about a patient using the mobile computers that are wheeled from room to room.

Bottom: Family Medicine Practitioner Dr. Andrew Coren listens to his patient's heartbeat. Dr. Coren remained in private practice for most of his career, long after most of his colleagues joined a medical group.

FAMILY MEDICINE RESIDENCY

Since the 1950s, when surgical specialists began earning higher wages for procedures than general practitioners earned for providing primary care, fewer and fewer doctors were attracted to primary care. The heirs to general practitioners were internists (who treat adults), pediatricians (who treat children), and family practitioners (who treat everyone).

After decades of higher reimbursements for procedures and the accompanying prestige that went with being a surgical specialist, a dramatic shortage of primary care doctors emerged, which was especially concerning given the number of baby boomers about to reach an age when they would need more health care.

In 2015, there were not enough primary care doctors for the population in Ukiah, and many of the doctors in the area were nearing retirement. Dr. Evans said of the UVMC service area, "We need forty-two primary care doctors, and we have twenty-eight—nine of whom are over sixty-five [years old]." This equated to approximately 40,000 people in the Ukiah area without a primary care doctor—people who, without adequate access to a doctor, often delayed care until they faced a medical emergency or their disease progressed to the point where treatment was no longer effective or available.

Ukiah has a history of creating educational opportunities to provide local people with the expertise to meet local needs. For example, in the 1990s, a Ukiah-based nursing program established to combat the national nursing shortage led to a successful source of nurses for the community. So, considering the shortage of primary care doctors, in 2015 a group of local primary care physicians led by Dr. Noemi "Mimi" Doohan, Dr. Lynne Coen, and Dr. Evans began working with Ukiah Valley Medical Center and the University of California at Davis to establish a family medicine residency program in the area. Statistics show that 75 percent of medical residents stay close to where they finish their training, so why not have some of them stay in the region?[30]

UVMC stepped forward as the institutional sponsor of the residency program and sought Adventist Health's support in doing so; this support was obtained May 9, 2015. Dr. Evans said, "The sum of the costs of program development over three years is estimated to be $1.5 million. At the end of the first year of the program (projected to be July 2019) we would then start receiving GME [graduate medical education] money from the federal government."

Dr. Evans also talked about the need for staff (a director and a coordinator), curriculum development, a residency practice center where residents can care for

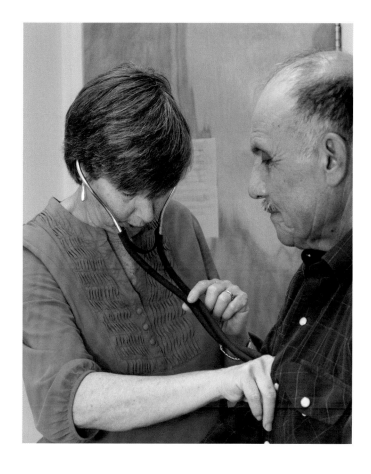

Family Medicine Practitioner Dr. Lynne Coen converses with her patient in Spanish while listening to his lungs.

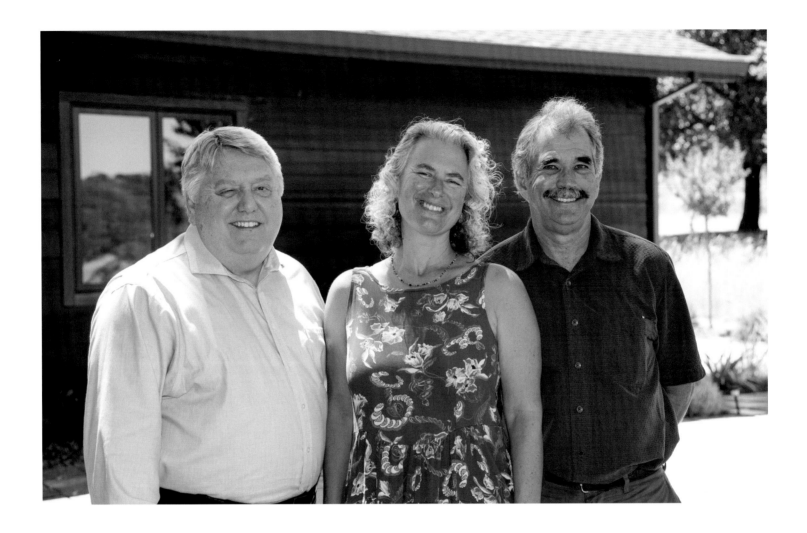

"It's going to be places like Ukiah that are going to teach us how to get back there [knowing and understanding patients], because we're fighting, in the urban settings, these incredible turf wars; it's like an arms race. Billboards say, 'Our hospital's got three MRIs.' 'Ours has seven.' "

patients, housing for the residents and their families, and figuring out the operations of the program—including rotations and scheduling. "There are so many facets to this," Dr. Evans explained.

With encouragement from Dr. Doohan, a community group called Family Medicine Education for Mendocino County (FMEMC) began fundraising as soon as they learned about the program. FMEMC is raising funds for the development phase of the program, as well as faculty education and training.

Dr. Evans said, "Physicians love to teach, but they don't love to teach to the detriment of feeding their families and sending their kids to school. There needs to be a give and take here—if you're going to give me twenty hours a month, we need to do something for you because that's twenty hours in the office that would have earned income."

Ukiah's budding commitment to this project garnered the attention of family medicine leaders outside of the area. Professor Richard Roberts, MD, JD, an internationally recognized champion of family medicine, said, "I think in many ways in the United States, we've come to think about health care as doing stuff to people rather than knowing them and understanding them and addressing their concerns. And that may seem like a small or even a silly thing, but I actually think it's fundamental to the problem.

"If we're going to get back to where I think we need to be in terms of a health care system that actually does that, it's going to be places like Ukiah that are going to teach us how to get back there, because we're fighting, in the urban settings, these incredible turf wars; it's like an arms race. Billboards say, 'Our hospital's got three MRIs.' 'Ours has seven.' And frankly, that is not only bad medical practice—because people are getting tests they don't need and it's terribly expensive—but it's iterative. It keeps escalating. And so, what we're proposing Ukiah can do is to help, be a shining example, show that it can be done right."

Dr. Doohan, family practitioner and lead author of *Back to the Future: Reflections on the History of the Future of Family Medicine*, has been a driving force in starting Ukiah's family medicine residency program. She believes family medicine is "uniquely positioned to lead efforts to help our nation achieve the triple aim of better health care, improved population health, and lower health care costs." She agrees with the recommendation of the Future

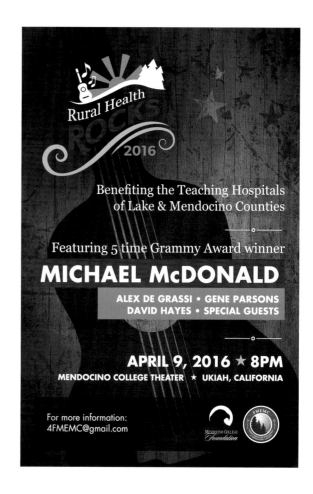

Above: Family Medicine Education for Mendocino County (FMEMC) hosted a benefit concert to raise funds for the family medicine residency program.

Opposite: Dr. Richard Roberts, Dr. Mimi Doohan, and Dr. Charlie Evans are working together to start a family medicine residency program in Ukiah.

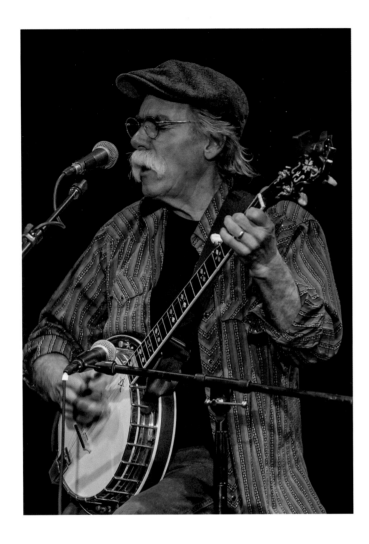

Gene Parsons strums his banjo at Rural Health Rocks, the 2016 benefit concert for Ukiah's family medicine residency program. Parsons, formerly of the Byrds, is the inventor of the Parsons White Stringbender, a device used by many rock musicians.

Family of Medicine project that the family medicine scope of practice should encompass a comprehensive approach to caring for the whole person, but she recognizes the difficulties of this approach.

"This has been challenging because of malpractice insurance, reimbursement, lifestyle priorities, credentialing, and lack of support from other medical specialists," she notes, but "at the same time, an increasing percentage of family physicians are engaged in comprehensive prevention and chronic illness management for individuals as well as caring for communities and populations, demonstrating that family medicine has expanded in complexity if not in scope."[31]

Dr. Doohan's hope is that starting a new family medicine residency program in Ukiah will not only provide the local population with desperately needed primary care physicians, but also, if done right, be a model for continuing to influence the direction of family medicine in the United States.

WHOLE-PERSON CARE IN UKIAH

The idea of whole-person care is not new, but rather a return to medicine's origins found in many healing traditions, including Ukiah's oldest: those of Pomo peoples.

The American Indian healers from local Pomo tribes, who were sometimes called "Dreamers," cared for the sick and ailing through songs and prayers as well as with poultices, tonics, and mementos infused with spiritual strength. Before European settlers came to the area, nearly all Pomo communities had ceremonial roundhouses, where healing ceremonies usually took place.

With the arrival of European settlers came new healing traditions, and as technology enabled the rapid spread of information, healing traditions from all over the world became refined, codified, and shared in varying degrees.

Regardless of tradition, the future of medicine should be guided by care that works best for the patient, defining clear goals for medical results and providing an experience that reduces stress and makes the patient feel as comfortable as possible, both physically and emotionally.

Today, even the most technologically advanced American hospitals seek to treat the whole person—body, mind, and spirit. It is seen as a best practice, and studies such as those by Harvard researcher Dr. Herbert Benson demonstrate the power of prayer and meditation in aiding the healing process.

As part of Adventist Health, Ukiah Valley Medical Center employs a full-time chaplain and invites spiritual leaders from the community, including Buddhist monks and nuns from the nearby City of Ten Thousand Buddhas, Catholic priests from Saint Mary of the Angels Catholic Church, and many others from Christian and non-Christian traditions to support patients who request a spiritual element to their care. In fact, the hospital's mission is to "reflect God's love by providing physical, mental, and spiritual healing."

While prayer and other spiritual practices have long brought ailing people comfort, until recently, hospitals rarely created soothing environments for patients. More commonly, hospital facilities offered an impersonal atmosphere dominated by technology, with white walls, stainless steel trays, and a focus on minimizing infection. Making a hospital feel more like home, creating an atmosphere more conducive to healing by employing calming colors, relaxing music, beautiful art, therapeutic massage, and aromatherapy as well as practical aids such as earplugs and eye shades has gained favor in recent decades with the popularity of national programs such as Planetree. According to their website, Planetree helps health care organizations create this improved atmosphere by offering "a structured methodology for humanizing, personalizing and demystifying the patient experience."

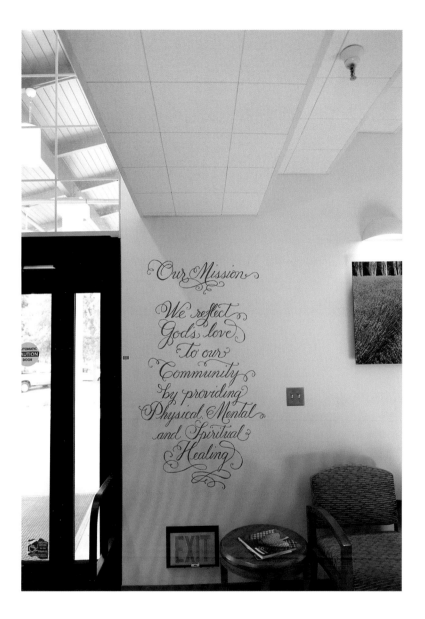

Ukiah Valley Medical Center uses artwork to create a peaceful, spiritual atmosphere. This mission statement graces the wall adjacent to the Family Birth Center entrance.

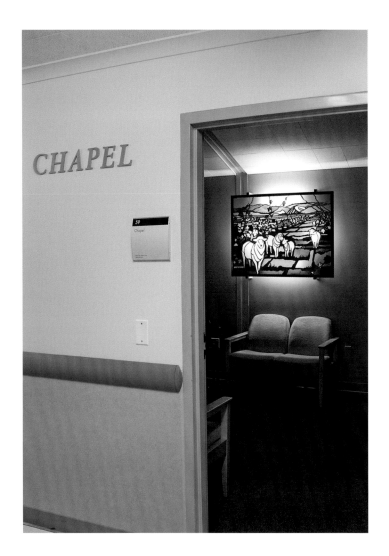

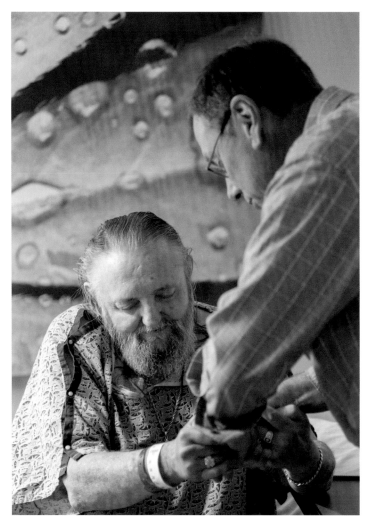

Left: Ukiah Valley Medical Center offers the use of its chapel to visitors for reflection, and sometimes for mourning.

Right: Patient William Kidd prays with Chaplain Mike Dobbs before surgery.

In a sense, it is as though health care has come full circle. When medicine could offer little more than prayer and comfort, the spiritual and emotional needs of patients were considered equal partners with medical technology.

In a sense, it is as though health care has come full circle. When medicine could offer little more than prayer and comfort, the spiritual and emotional needs of patients were considered equal partners with medical technology. As scientific breakthroughs gave the medical community confidence that it could eventually conquer almost any illness, more people received care in hospitals, which were designed with technology and intervention—rather than comfort—as a top priority. In 2016, at least in Ukiah, hospitals and health centers have embraced the blending of a soothing environment with highly advanced care that attends to the body, mind, and spirit.

Looking to the future, the hospital is working with Delos, a company dedicated to creating built environments that promote healthy indoor living. UVMC is hoping to work with Delos to modify its WELL Building Standard so it can be implemented for health care buildings. The current standard seeks to assure that a built environment promotes human health and wellness by focusing on air, water, nourishment, light, fitness, comfort, and mind. This is good for patients and visitors and also for those who spend the most time in hospitals: the employees, allied health staff, and medical staff.

Regardless of how comfortable patients are made and how advanced technology becomes, modern medicine will never be able to address all of the diseases and failings of the human body. Death is inevitable, and if physical, mental, and spiritual health are truly to be provided, consideration must be given to how people are helped into and out of this world.

During the last forty years, a revolution of sorts has occurred in the way doctors approach birthing care, from the 1970s, when women were shaved, strapped to stirrups, and often rushed

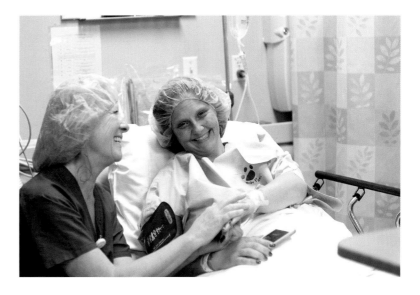

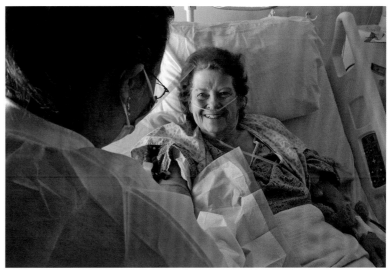

Top: Nurse Nancy Bray, RN, smiles at patient Natalie Shepard before surgery.

Bottom: Patient Kittie Hawk says Avelina "Lina" Pottinger, her dialysis nurse, is her "angel."

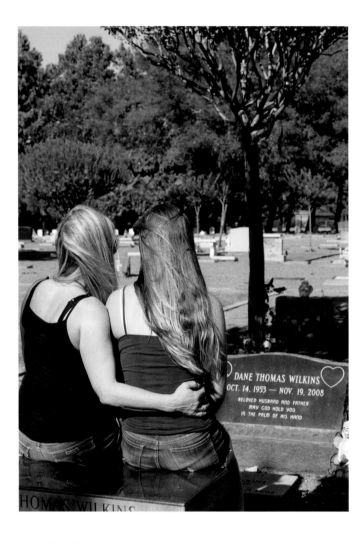

Widow Elise Wilkins, RN, hugs her daughter while they pay their respects to husband and father Dane Wilkins, former Ukiah Valley Medical Center Respiratory Therapy Director.

along with Pitocin to the 2010s, when modern hospitals allow water births, obstetricians work with certified nurse midwives, and women are given choices about how much medication to use for pain and birth progression.

The same revolution has begun with end-of-life care, and the Ukiah community is embracing this change. While everyone can agree that death is inevitable, we still have a difficult time letting go. We celebrate birth. We care for the young and teach them to become self-sufficient adults. And we admire older adults who remain strong, but as frailty sets in and people are less able to care for themselves, most of us are ill equipped to handle the situation, physically or emotionally.

We seem to have adopted poet Dylan Thomas' plea in *Do not go gentle into that good night*. We rage against the dying of the light. According to author Dr. Atul Gawande in his bestselling book *Being Mortal: Medicine and What Matters in the End*, American medicine has an important shift to undertake if we are to help people experience peaceful, natural deaths.

Health care professionals are in a unique position to learn, and then help the rest of us learn, how to have conversations about dying rather than ignoring the subject until it is too painful or too late to comply with a person's dying wishes.

Toward that end, the hospice movement has made great strides. Hospice care is end-of-life care, and its evolution in Ukiah has been due, in great part, to the efforts of family practitioner Dr. Robert Werra.

Hospice Care

Traditionally, hospitals were made up of long wards with beds lining the walls and a chapel at the end. When nothing more could be done for a patient, he or she was put at the end of the row in a bed closest to the chapel. Eventually, chapels were replaced by more beds. Dr. Werra shared what happened when modern medicine had nothing left to offer patients.

When I was in medical school, we went to the county hospital and we went to the veterans' hospital, and the hospitals were all kind of the same. When we would make rounds, there would be the chief doctor and then the resident and then the intern and then the nurse, and we'd go from bed to bed and make rounds and discuss each case each morning, then decide what needed to be done.

And what happened was, people who you couldn't cure anymore or fix anymore (because in medicine, our job is to fix people, and so if we couldn't fix them anymore, we didn't know what to do)—they were put down at the end.

Then, when we would make rounds, we would go down to the end and then skip over to the other side because there wasn't anything to do for those people.

There was no training in medical school on how to take care of people when you couldn't fix them anymore, and like all humans, when you don't know something, you go into denial or ignore it. It wasn't a conscious thing.

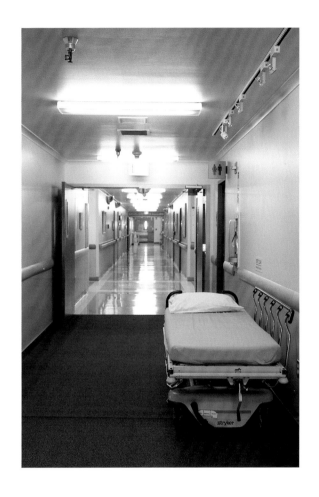

Because doctors are traditionally trained to "fix" people, it is hard to know how to provide care and comfort when patients are terminally ill.

In the 1960s, doctors commonly gave Demerol injections to reduce pain for the terminally ill, but by today's standards, doctors waited too long—until patients were clearly in distress—to give it. Oral pain medication was a breakthrough for end-of-life care because it made administering the medication so much easier on the patient; eventually, medication was given often enough so it would stay in the patient's system and provide better around-the-clock comfort. But giving Demerol to numb the pain was not enough to provide an emotionally satisfying end-of-life experience.

The term *hospice* can trace its roots back to the Crusades. A hospice was a "rest house" or refuge for religious pilgrims, a place of hospitality. It became associated with end-of-life care thanks to the pioneering work of British nurse-turned-doctor Dame Cicely Saunders, who believed end-of-life care should address what she called "total pain" (physical, emotional, social, and spiritual pain). She founded St. Christopher's Hospice in London and that inspired Dr. Werra to follow her lead, so much so that Dr. Werra visited St. Christopher's in the early 2000s (only to find that Dr.

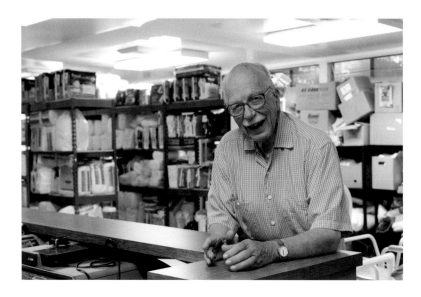

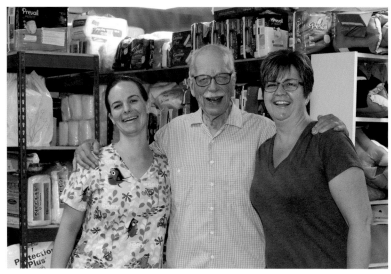

Top: Family Medicine Practitioner Dr. Robert Werra tells one of his many stories while spending time at the hospice he helped create.

Bottom: Hospice of Ukiah workers are not beholden to federal funds and can therefore be more flexible in the way they provide treatment and care. Left to right: Suzanne Pollesel, Home Health Aid, Dr. Robert Werra, Diane Keeton, LVN.

Opposite: Providing end-of-life care at home instead of at a hospital allows patients to remain more comfortable in their final weeks.

Saunders was no longer the medical director, but was now a patient receiving the very care she helped champion).

In the late 1970s, hospice care jumped across the pond, moving from the United Kingdom to the United States. During that move, Americans changed hospice from a facility-based endeavor to a volunteer service that supported patients so they could die peacefully at home.

By 1980, hospice services were "springing up like wildflowers all over our country," Dr. Werra said. Hospitals started them. The Visiting Nurses Association started them. People in communities all over the country started them, inspiring Dr. Werra and others in Ukiah to hold a town meeting to see if Ukiah should have one. Dr. Werra and Mendocino College drama teacher Bob Alto invited community members to the Mendocino College Little Theater back when the college was located at the Redwood Empire Fairgrounds. Alto chaired the meeting, and he and Dr. Werra, who was the only physician present, asked if people would be interested in having a hospice service in Ukiah. The general consensus was a resounding yes.

Shortly thereafter, a small group of hospice enthusiasts invited Dr. Werra to meet so they could share their specific ideas about who hospice would help and how. They had plans to provide emotional support, nutritional support, and other end-of-life care, and they asked Dr. Werra if he would be the hospice medical director.

"So we were talking about it, and their concept was, 'We're going to save people from the pain and misery of radiation and chemotherapy. We'll save them from the doctors. And they're going to accept dying, and we're going to make dying pleasant for them, and we'll get them out of the hands of the doctors,'" Dr. Werra said.

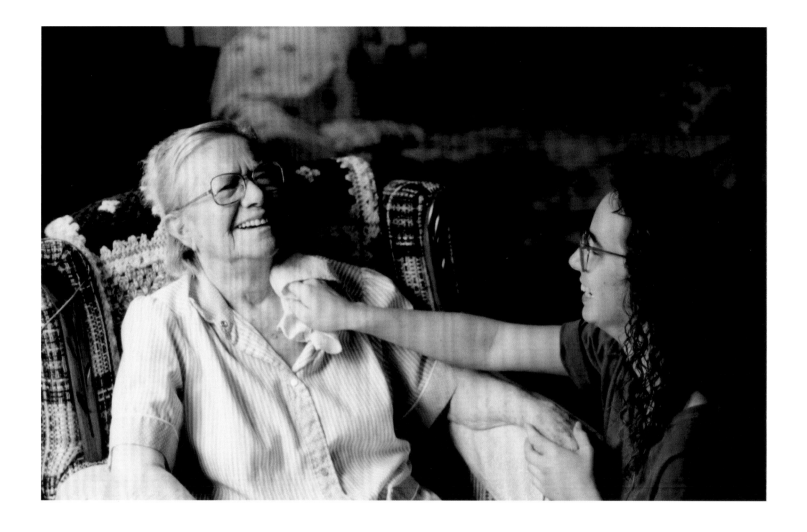

In the late 1970s, hospice care jumped across the pond, moving from the United Kingdom to the United States. During that move, Americans changed hospice from a facility-based endeavor to a volunteer service that supported patients so they could die peacefully at home.

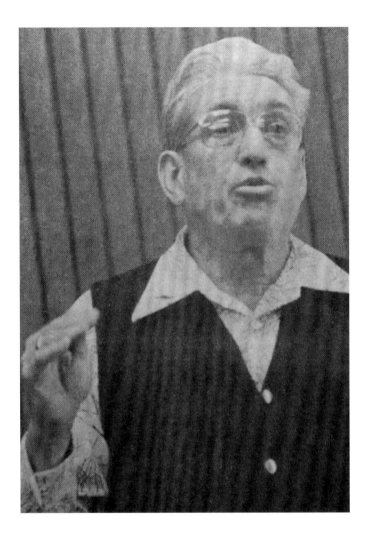

Burt Banzhaf collaborated with Dr. Robert Werra to provide hospice services in Ukiah.

Although Dr. Werra was a doctor himself, he was not offended. He understood why people wanted to avoid the side effects of radiation and chemotherapy, and he did not deny the medical community's penchant for intervention at the end of life. However, he worried that no doctor he knew would refer patients to this voluntary hospice service, given the doctors' training to fix, fix, fix.

"If we're going to have this, who's going to refer patients? Is a doctor going to refer to this quacky business? I don't think this is going to work," he thought. But he believed in it and he supported it, and eventually, other doctors did, too.

A few years earlier, Medicare had begun funding home nursing visits and Ukiah had a fledgling home health agency with Dr. Werra as its medical director. Since it seemed clear that the community wanted a hospice service, Dr. Werra asked the Mendocino Home Health agency director, Burt Banzhaf, if Hospice of Ukiah—as they were calling themselves—might work under the auspices of the Home Health agency. Banzhaf was receptive, so Dr. Werra invited hospice pioneer and former medical school classmate Dr. William Lamers to Ukiah to share his expertise and encouragement. "He brought his Kodak carousel slide projector and showed us slides about hospice. And I said to myself, 'We can do it,'" Dr. Werra said. And before they knew it, Ukiahans had a hospice service.

Very quickly, the benefits of hospice care became clear. While many people chose to combat death until the very end with traditional medical treatment, others opted for what they considered to be a more natural approach with hospice. And when medicine had nothing left to offer, hospice was ready with open arms. People who received hospice care and their families and friends shared their good hospice experiences in the community: less fear, more control, less pain, more lucidity and connectedness. And hospice grew.

Hospice services all over the country were gaining popularity, and after a landmark study by insurance company Aetna showed that hospice care helped people live longer with a better quality of life while costing health insurance companies less, the movement caught the eye of the federal government. In 1982, seeing the financial savings of less intervention at the end of life (when medical care is often most expensive), Medicare agreed to fund hospice care. However, as with most federal funding, strict rules applied. The founders of Hospice of Ukiah believed some of the rules would limit their service in unacceptable ways, so they opted to continue as a volunteer organization and forego federal funding.

As hospice rules continued to expand, a bill introduced in the California Senate threatened to limit the legal use of the word "hospice" to those organizations certified by Medicare, inspiring Dr. Werra and others in Mendocino County to write letters to California Senator Barry Keene, protesting this. Keene invited these constituents to his office, and after Dr. Werra's articulate and impassioned plea, Keene amended the legislation to allow Ukiah, Fort Bragg, Garberville, Willits, and Gualala to continue operating on a voluntary basis using the term *hospice.*

To be certified by Medicare—and therefore be eligible for federal funding—hospice services could care only for patients who were within six months of dying (as certified by their physician) and who agreed to forego medical intervention to prolong life. While this may seem reasonable, predicting the end of life is often more art than science, and requiring families to face the fact that their loved one was that close to death put hospice out of reach for many until it was too late.

As a volunteer organization with only a few health care professionals and limited staff, the organization could not provide services such as skilled nursing and around-the-clock availability. However, the dedicated team included nurses, a nutritionist, behavioral health professionals, clergy, and others who provided vital support to those facing death.

About a year after Hospice of Ukiah began, Medicare called the Home Health agency and asked whether they were doing hospice work out of their office. "Yes," they said. "A volunteer hospice." But Medicare argued that the hospice workers were benefiting from federal funding (electricity to run the office, rent on the office space, etc.), and therefore, the hospice service had to be certified under its rules.

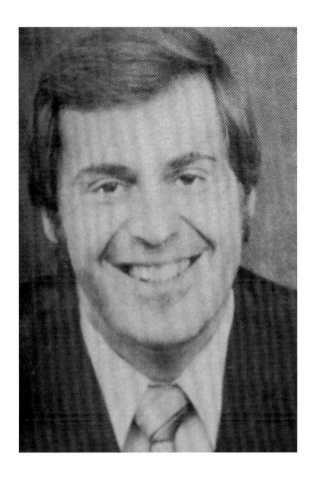

With encouragement from Dr. Robert Werra, California Senator Barry Keene provided the necessary support to allow the word "hospice" to be used for organizations outside the Medicare system.

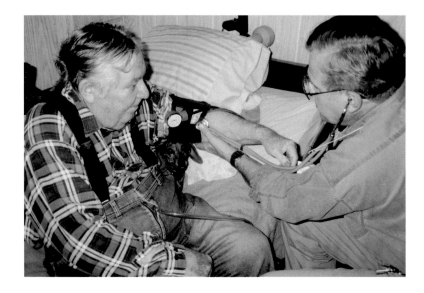

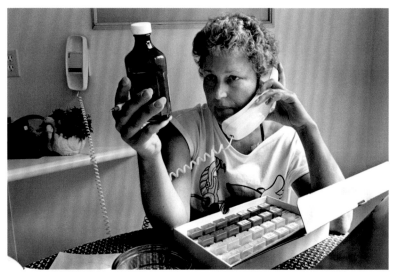

With support from doctors and nurses, people can receive care from family members and loved ones at the end of life.

Top: The patient's vital signs are taken and his catheter is checked to keep him safe and comfortable.

Bottom: A woman calls about medications to make sure she has what she needs.

As a result, hospice care in Ukiah split in two. Hospice of Ukiah moved out of the Home Health office and continued to provide volunteer hospice services. It eventually expanded to include palliative care, Alzheimer's care, and caregiver respite care; and Medicare-approved Phoenix Hospice accepted federal funding that allowed them to provide skilled nursing, case management, and twenty-four-hour availability to their patients. Both organizations continue to provide important end-of-life care for local patients.

Although doctors did not start the hospice movement, and in fact, were brought in "kicking and screaming," according to Dr. Werra, many have embraced the idea that less is more when it comes to medical intervention at the end of life, and they commonly refer patients to Ukiah's hospice services.

The success of hospice services gave rise to a broader movement, one that also focuses on comfort rather than cure: the palliative care movement. Palliative care is often provided at the end of life, but it is not limited to end-of-life care. While hospice care is for those within six months of dying, palliative care is for those within ten years of dying. Palliative care focuses on improving the quality of life for people facing debilitating illnesses. The term *palliative* is from the Latin root *pallium*, meaning to mask or cloak; palliative care, then, seeks to mask the pain. It uses a team approach to address physical and emotional pain and stress while providing spiritual support for those who want it.

A palliative care team is composed of a medical provider, a social worker, a nurse, a spiritual leader, and others. Ukiah Valley Medical Center's palliative care team also includes a speech pathologist because swallowing becomes difficult at the end of life, and sometimes the team includes volunteers who offer to sit with patients who would otherwise be alone in the hospital because they have no family or friends to be with them.

In Ukiah during the 2010s, the understanding of and appreciation for palliative care has grown dramatically. Palliative care has gone from a term few people recognized to a well-established service people know about and request. Palliative care employees and volunteers work in partnership with hospitals, hospice services, in-home health care, nursing homes, rehabilitation centers, senior centers, cancer treatment centers, and individual families.

According to physician assistant Lynn Meadows, leader of the UVMC Palliative Care team, the end-of-life conversation is what palliative care is about. "It is the basis of palliative care; you talk to your patients and find out what their wishes are. What a concept! Do you think we were trained in medical school to talk to our patients about this? No. So it's a revolution in health care in our country right now."

She refers to Dr. Atul Gawande's book, *Being Mortal*, and animatedly explains that the Boston-based author has developed a system for having the end-of-life conversation—referred to simply as "the conversation"—and collects data and teaches people to help the dying and their families in a unified way. "It's a nationwide thing we're going to be a part of at Ukiah Valley Medical Center," Meadows said. She was excited to share that she was one of twenty people nationwide to attend a training seminar taught by Dr. Gawande in 2015.

Palliative care workers are trained to lead family meetings about a dying loved one, starting with open-ended invitations to talk about the family's situation. While Meadows is informal by nature—preferring sandals and loose-fitting clothes to a starched white lab coat—she understands the delicate emotional state families are

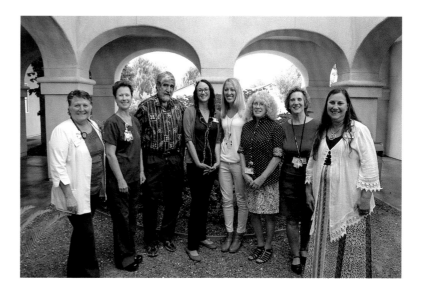

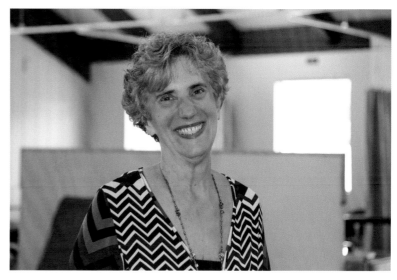

Top: Ukiah Valley Medical Center's Palliative Care Team helps patients and their families have the best experience possible at the end of life in accordance with their beliefs and wishes.

Bottom: When patients can no longer swallow properly at the end of life, speech pathologist Susan Pollesel helps families understand that the patient is declining and not expected to recover. Broaching the subject of death and dying is difficult, but it allows families to have a better end-of-life experience.

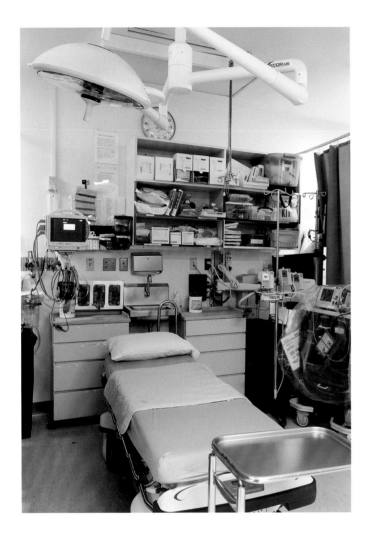

Physician assistant Lynn Meadows tries to help patients and their families understand that doing everything to sustain life at the very end of life can be intrusive and painful. If at all possible, she suggests, this emergency room bay is not where people should spend their last moments.

in when a loved one is dying. She described going to a family's house.

"I wear a white coat and use good posture when I go in there, and I say, 'Hi, I'm Lynn Meadows and I'm a PA and I'm here to help you.' And then I start with an open-ended question like, 'Tell me what you think is going on here.' Oh my gosh, the stuff that comes out of their mouths. It's amazing. It's like I said, 'I give you permission to speak the truth.'"

Families invariably begin sharing what they all know but are afraid to admit to themselves or each other, and the relief of admitting that death is coming helps people figure out how to best use the time that remains. Meadows said most people want to spend more time with family, remain at home, and want to have peace. "They want to sit on their deck in the sun or be surrounded by grandkids," she said. She emphasized that people do not want to be in the hospital being poked and prodded "for nothing," as she put it.

Meadows explained what happens in hospitals when a patient stops breathing (unless the patient has let it be known that he or she wants to be allowed to peacefully die a natural death). Medical providers begin chest compressions to see if they can restart a patient's heart; chest compressions often cause broken ribs. Medical providers then put a tube down the patient's throat to ventilate the lungs. For a person in the best of health, these activities are uncomfortable. For those at the end of life, whose bodies are frail and failing, these activities ruin the last moments of life.

She said, "That's what we do in America. That's death in America right now. Do you know how many people with serious illness survive CPR? Less than 1 percent. People need to be supported to go home and have spiritual care and loving care and nursing care."

Meadows spoke passionately about her frustration over the Medicare rules that limit hospice care to the last six months of life and require people to stop accepting life-prolonging treatment in favor of comfort care, because she knows that if people have to give up on life and welcome death to receive benefits, they will not do so until the last possible moment.

Meadows lamented the way people often use hospice care, calling it "too little, too late." According to a Medicare Payment Advisory Committee (MedPAC) report dated March 2014, most Medicare patients use hospice services for about seventeen days. A quarter of patients receive hospice care for a week or less, and about 10 percent use hospice services only in the last two to three days of life.

The change in end-of-life care Meadows described requires tools and training, and these are now being developed and shared. Hospitals are replacing Do Not Resuscitate (DNR) orders with Accept Natural Death (AND) orders. Physicians are working with patients to complete Physician Orders for Life-Sustaining Treatment (POLST) forms so patients' wishes about medical treatment at the end of life can be honored. And most importantly, medical providers are learning how to have the conversation to help patients and their families embrace the time they have left.

As with other facets of health care, end-of-life care continues to evolve; just as the human body constantly seeks homeostasis, so too, over time, has medicine sought to find the right balance between intervention and comfort. The goal, of course, is to create ways to help people live full, healthy, productive lives and die peacefully in accordance with their wishes and beliefs.

The evolution of end-of-life care is one of many examples of how medicine is integrating technology while ensuring that a patient's overall experience is as comforting as possible.

The Physician Orders for Life-Sustaining Treatment (POLST) form allows doctors to review end-of-life preferences with patients.

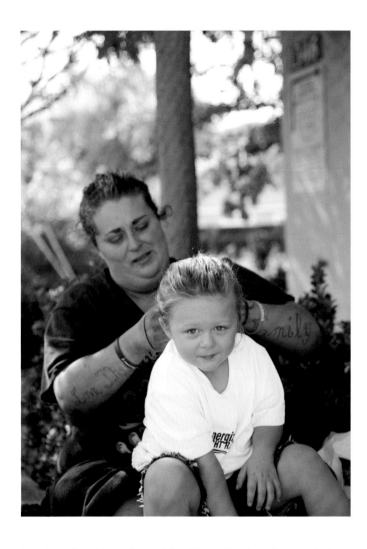

A mother pulls back her son's hair while waiting for Plowshares Peace and Justice Center of Ukiah to open in 2015.

STREET MEDICINE

The last frontier of medicine may be the streets, going to the homeless and disenfranchised and meeting them where they are, physically and emotionally. Nationally recognized street medicine pioneer Dr. Jim Withers visited Ukiah in October 2015 to see one of his protégés, Dr. Mimi Doohan, and to meet with community members to help Dr. Doohan garner support for a rural street medicine program. Dr. Withers defined street medicine as "honoring and engaging the reality of excluded people," adding that another name for street medicine is "inclusion health."

Dr. Doohan sees Ukiah as fertile soil in which to plant a robust rural street medicine program, which would be among the first rural teaching hospital-affiliated programs in the nation. (Currently, only a few metropolitan areas have organized street medicine programs.) Dr. Doohan successfully started a program in Santa Barbara in 2005, which is still growing and thriving. She is currently helping to start two other street medicine programs in the Palm Springs area.

Dr. Doohan sees special potential in Ukiah. "Ukiah is different," she explained. "Here you've got mature, open organizations coming forward and saying, 'We're really stretched thin, but if we can work together somehow, let's do it.' People here are very open about what their concerns are and what their strengths are. So we've applied for a grant to build on the strengths that already exist by creating resources that help connect these organizations to each other."

The spread of street medicine is music to Dr. Withers' ears. He began reaching out and caring for the homeless in Pittsburgh, Pennsylvania, in the 1990s, and by incorporating medical students into his street practice and giving lectures all over the country and the world, he has helped ignite a movement. "We're saving ourselves," he explained. This "reality-based" health care transcends the bureaucratic medical system and allows clinicians who originally followed a calling to return to that calling.

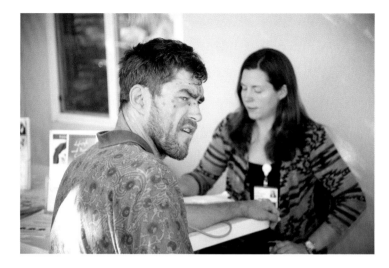

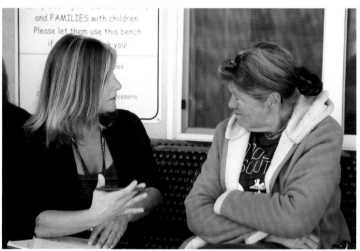

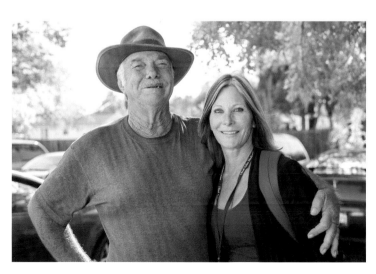

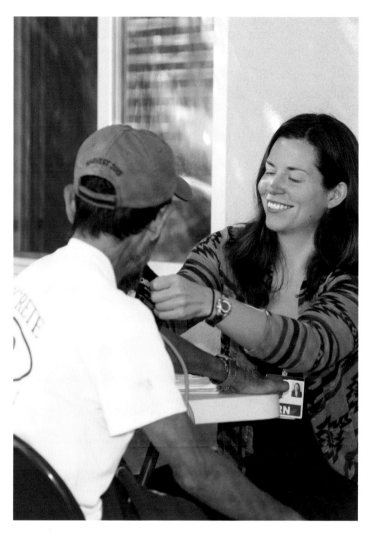

Leanna Sweet, RN, (top and right), and Wellness Coach Michelle Flowers (middle and bottom) offer health check-ups and education for people in line to receive free meals from Plowshares Peace and Justice Center of Ukiah.

"No matter how mistreated or excluded someone is, no matter who they are, they still have a certain level of assumed trust and respect for the person who is caring for their health, and that's at stake. If we don't live up to that in spirit as well as technology, then we're in trouble," he said. The thing that baffles Dr. Withers as well as Dr. Doohan is the attitude that they are somehow saints to be doing this work when they believe it should be the norm. Dr. Withers described how he feels:

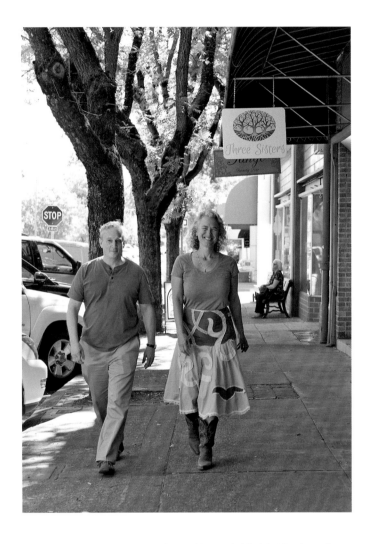

Street medicine pioneer Dr. Jim Withers and his protégé Dr. Mimi Doohan walk down School Street during Dr. Withers' visit to Ukiah.

I know that what I thought was an impossible dream and a leap of faith resulted in a small group of people, homeless themselves, and then others—nurses and such—saying, "We're in this together." And I've watched that spirit grow and grow. We have a global movement now.

Fear, negativity, division—they are strong, fast, powerful forces. Unity and love are slower but they are stronger, and we know that in our hearts. And if we just don't give up and we stay together, they prevail, because we really do, in the deepest sense, want to heal ourselves. I've watched it happen, and I have a lot of faith that it's a matter of staying the course.

People will exploit those fast, short-term, negative things to build false community in which people agree on whom they hate to feel closer to each other, but it's never satisfying, and it never solves any problems. The only way we solve problems is to treat others the way we want to be treated and demand that that's who we are. I think health care is just one arena for that, but it is intrinsically charged with caring about each other, so it's a natural and powerful ally in that deeper vision.

Ukiah Valley Medical Center agrees with this vision and has put its full support behind Dr. Doohan to help her create the type of street medicine program that reaches out to the patients who do not engage in the health system if it requires them to enter a doctor's office, medical clinic, or hospital. A small team from the hospital has been visiting Plowshares, an organization dedicated to feeding the poor, and providing basic health care to those who are interested. This helps to lay the groundwork for a full street medicine program.

The goal of the street medicine program is to connect people with the resources to address the social determinants of health, including having a primary care provider with whom the full resources of modern medicine can be brought to bear. But initially, medical care in a shelter or on the streets is better than no care, and offering acceptance and kindness is potent medicine in and of itself. Hospital president Gwen Matthews shared the story of the Cassell brothers to illustrate this kind of medicine.

THE CONNECTEDNESS OF MEDICINE

Randy Cassell lived on the streets for much of his life, abusing drugs and running afoul of the law. He was brought to UVMC from Lake County because his cancer had progressed to a point that he required specialized care. By the time he was hospitalized, his days were numbered. When a pastor who had befriended him asked if he had any family, Cassell responded that he had a brother, Scott, with whom he had not been in touch since Cassell was a teen. Cassell told the pastor that he thought his brother was a famous oceanographer. Instead of dismissing Cassell as delusional, the pastor investigated Cassell's assertion and found an accomplished deep-sea diver named Scott Cassell online. The pastor got in touch with Scott and asked if he had a brother named Randy. Scott confirmed that he did but had not seen him in years.

The Cassell brothers grew up with an abusive father. In his early teens, Randy defied his father to save his mother—running to the neighbors to call an ambulance after his father assaulted her. It was the point of no return; Randy could never go back home. Thus began his life on the streets. When Scott Cassell came to the

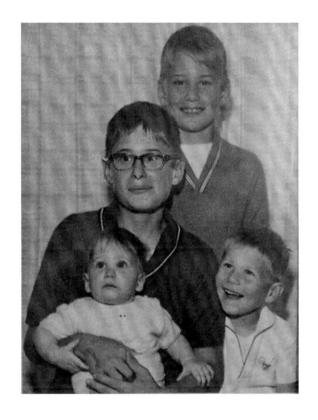

The Cassell brothers grew up with an abusive father. When Randy Cassell (standing) protected his mother, he was cast out of the house at age fourteen. He didn't spend time with his brother Scott (lower right) until the end of Randy's life, and only then because of the kindness of health care professionals in Ukiah.

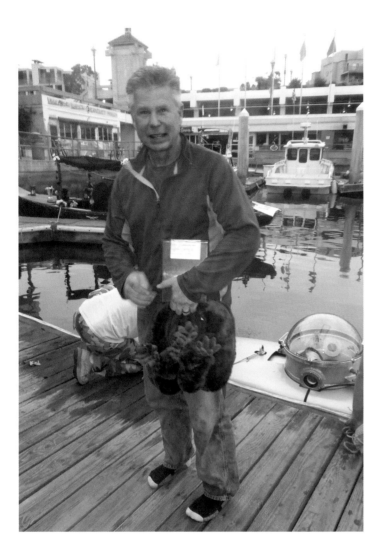

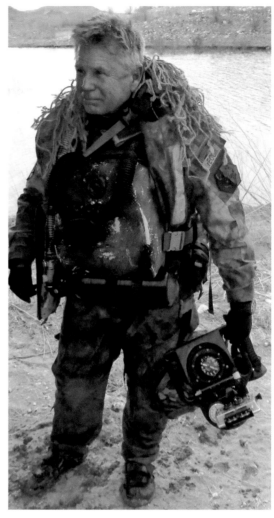

Left: Scott Cassell holds his brother Randy's ashes and prepares to take them into the ocean as part of his maiden voyage in his submarine, the Great White.

Right: As an oceanographer, Scott Cassell founded the Undersea Voyager Project, an organization dedicated to advancing scientific knowledge about marine life and educating youth.

Here was a famous oceanographer meeting his hero: his homeless brother with a law enforcement tracking device around his ankle. The healing for both of them was profound.

hospital, he told his brother that Randy had always been his hero for saving their mother's life. Here was a famous oceanographer meeting his hero: his homeless brother with a law enforcement tracking device around his ankle. The healing for both of them was profound. Randy's cancer would end his life, but not before hospital and law enforcement staff went out of their way to make Randy's last wish come true: to see the ocean with his brother.

According to Scott Cassell's wife, Kerry, the nurses involved learned that Randy liked music by Sammy Hagar, so they bought him a CD that they all listened to on the way to the coast.

Matthews said, "You know, the purpose of health care hasn't changed through the years. It's just that now we have more diverse approaches." She praised the courage of people in health care to tackle the tough problems and shared her fervent belief that real and lasting change comes when people band together.

She said, "When I first arrived in Ukiah, I said, 'Wow, people here really care deeply about issues that affect their community.' While this has led to rifts in the past, it is also what makes the future so hopeful."

Matthews believes health care is at a tipping point, that it is blending old wisdom with new knowledge so that passion and skill can converge to deliver the extraordinary. "It's happening in Ukiah. I can feel it. I can't wait to see what the future holds," she said.

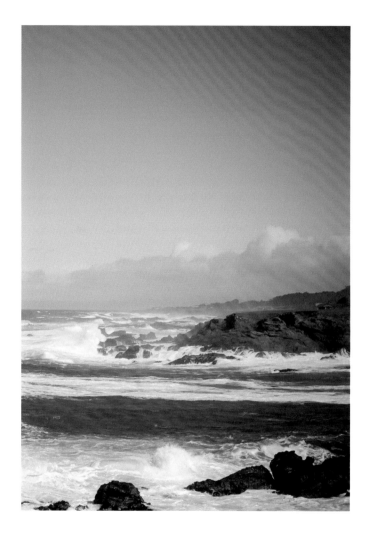

Above: The Cassell brothers were able to see the Mendocino Coast together before Randy's demise.

Next Page: Theresa Lund, RN, updates a patient chart before electronic medical records.

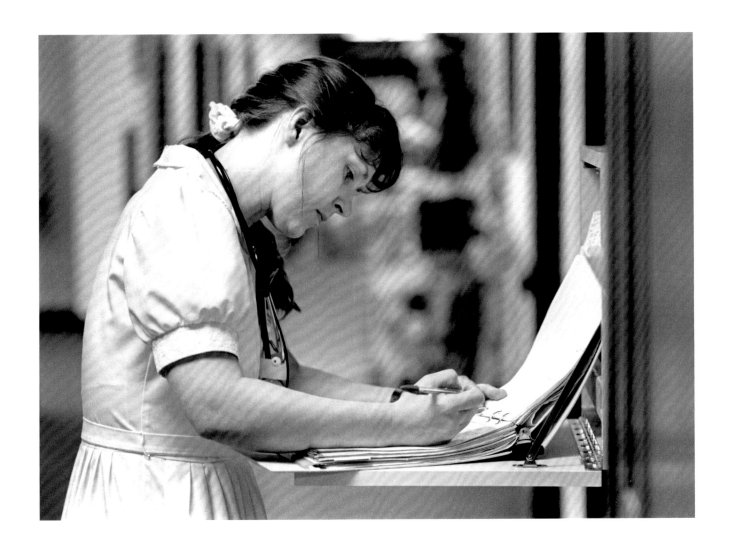

"After almost forty years in health care working in a variety of settings, from big teaching hospitals to small community hospitals, I can say without reservation that I have had the privilege of working with some of the finest people anywhere here in Ukiah."

–Gwen Matthews, President and CEO, Ukiah Valley Medical Center

AFTERWORD

After almost forty years in health care working in a variety of settings, from big teaching hospitals to small community hospitals, I can say without reservation that I have had the privilege of working with some of the finest people anywhere here in Ukiah.

Through this seminal period of great change in the way health care is paid for and the way it is delivered, we have created new ways to forge partnerships to improve the health of people in our community. We have worked together to plan for the future, laying a strong foundation in our built environment with the opening of our new ER and ICU as well as in laying out the whole campus expansion plan that will make UVMC a hub of wellness, not just a place to care for the sick.

We have also laid a strong foundation to ensure we have physicians available in our rural communities by developing a family medicine training program that will welcome its first residents in the summer of 2018.

These residents will have the opportunity to experience first-hand what it means to participate in a "community of solution" as well as the new era models of health care. They will learn from us how to innovate and how to design their own destinies.

Dodinsky, author of the New York Times bestseller *In The Garden of Thoughts*, said it so well: "Look not at the days gone by with a forlorn heart. They were simply the dots we can now connect with our present to help us draw the outline of a beautiful tomorrow."

Here's to all who have gone before and all who will forge new paths into the future to fulfill our mission to share God's love with our community by providing physical, mental, and spiritual healing. I truly believe the best is yet to come!

Gwen Matthews, RN, MSc, MBA
President and CEO, Ukiah Valley Medical Center

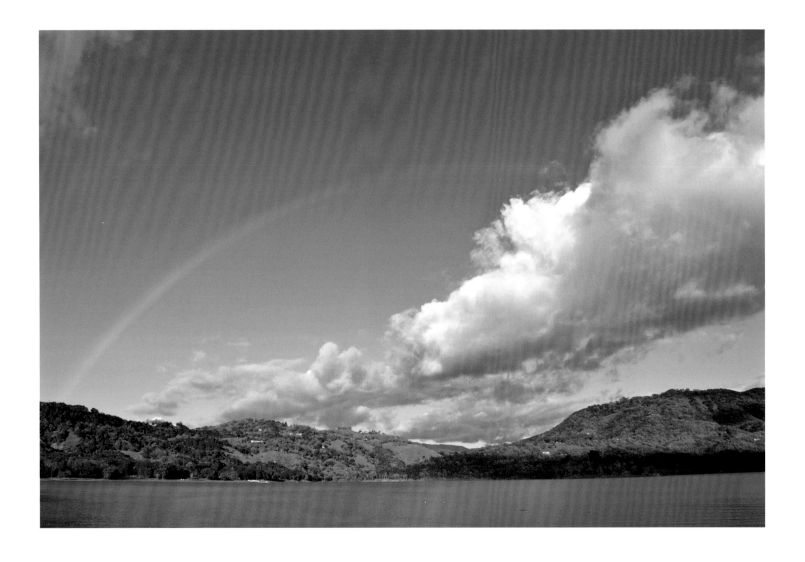

Decisions meant to solve a problem, such as improving access or increasing efficiency for one population, often created unforeseen consequences for other populations.

APPENDIX A

The Law of Unintended Consequences

The United States has the most expensive health care system in the world but by no means the best outcomes. We spend about 17 percent of our gross domestic product (GDP) on health care, while France and Sweden, ranked next, spend 11.6 percent and 11.5 percent, respectively. Out of eleven developed countries, the United States ranks dead last in efficiency, equity, and healthy lives. The United States did, however, rate in the top five for effectiveness of care, patient-centered care, and timeliness of care.

The way health care is delivered in America has largely been shaped by the way it has been paid for. During the last few decades, the government, as well as insurance health plans, have paid on a fee-for-service basis that resulted in a focus on discrete episodes of care rather than considering health care as a whole, interconnected, interdependent system. The more visits, the more tests, the more hospitalizations, the more the providers of health care got paid; however, there was no guarantee that the outcomes were improved.

Decisions meant to solve a problem, such as improving access or increasing efficiency for one population, often created unforeseen consequences for other populations. For example, paying more for highly trained surgeons to perform complex procedures encouraged many doctors to specialize to the point of causing a scarcity of primary care doctors. No one was paying much for prevention and health education, as the long-term benefits might not be realized if a patient changed health plans. When no one is paying for these upstream services, guess what happens? Very little. And people who were already paying health care premiums were not willing to pay out-of-pocket for things like cardiac rehabilitation.

Author Dr. Atul Gawande addresses this issue beautifully in his *New Yorker* piece titled "Overkill," in which he discusses the implications of over-testing.[32] He uses cancer screening as an example, explaining that through mammography, ultrasound, and blood tests, many more patients have been diagnosed and treated for breast cancer, thyroid cancer, and prostate cancer.

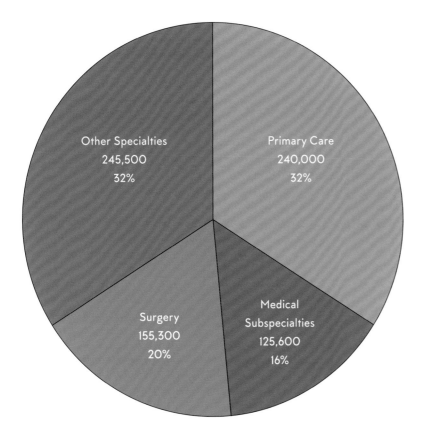

Ratios of Primary Care & Specialties

As of 2013, the distribution of active physicians shows increasing numbers of physicians pursuing specialty care due to current funding trends that encourage specialization. This bias toward specialty care is a significant contributing factor to the growing shortage of primary care physicians as shown in the chart on the facing page.

Primary Care includes general and family medicine, general internal medicine, general pediatrics, and geriatric medicine.

Medical Subspecialties include allergy and immunology, cardiology, critical care, dermatology, endocrinology, gastroenterology, hematology and oncology, infectious diseases, neonatal-perinatal medicine, nephrology, pulmonology, and rheumatology.

Surgery includes general surgery, colorectal surgery, neurological surgery, obstetrics and gynecology, ophthalmology, orthopedic surgery, otolaryngology, plastic surgery, thoracic surgery, urology, and vascular surgery.

Other Specialties includes anesthesiology, emergency medicine, neurology, pathology, physical medicine and rehabilitation, psychiatry, and radiology, among others.

"We're treating hundreds of thousands more people each year for these diseases than we ever have. Yet only a tiny reduction in death, if any, has resulted," he says.

Here is the problem: when we or one of our loved ones gets sick, we want doctors to do everything they can to understand and fix the problem. As Steven Brill writes in his book *America's Bitter Pill: Money, Politics, Backroom Deals, and the Fight to Fix Our Broken Healthcare System*, to him, the MRI had represented much of what was wrong with American health care: an often unnecessary and always expensive test that did little to improve most people's health. That is, until that very test identified his aortic embolism; "now the MRI was the miraculous lifesaver that found...the bomb hiding in my chest."

So where do we go from here? The good news is that modern health care decision-making is attempting to correct the unintended consequences of decades of piecemeal thinking. The Centers for Medicare and Medicaid Services (CMS) recognized this at the turn of the twenty-first century and started the Pay for Performance program, which began by refusing to pay hospitals for complications of care that happened during a hospitalization. This included any infections the patient acquired while in the hospital, injuries from patient falls, and surgical complications. Pay for Performance developed the core measures for high-volume hospital admissions, rewarding those hospitals that complied with evidence-based care and penalizing those that did not. Extension of coverage was made possible through the Affordable Care Act—a bold and welcome change, but only the beginning. Those who have benefited from the health care system as it has been will fight change; lobbyists continue to be incredibly influential.

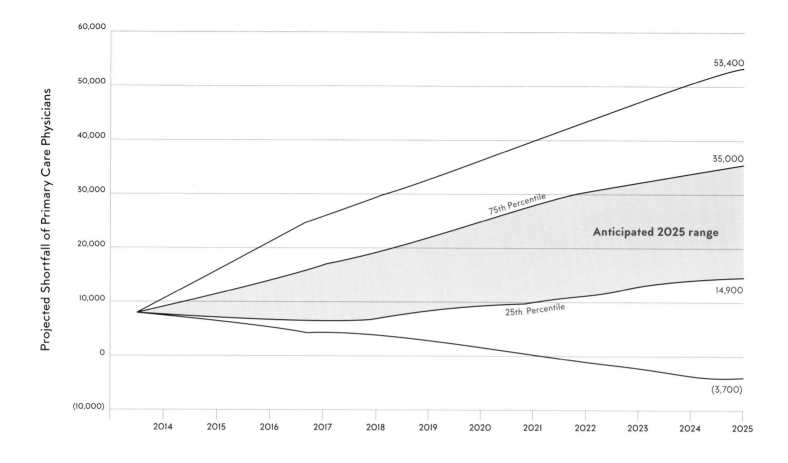

The Shortage of Primary Care Physicians

By the year 2025, projections indicate the US will experience a shortage between 14,900 and 35,600 primary care doctors. The above model is based on several scenarios that consider various combinations of factors, including the age at which physicians will retire (more than one-third of all currently active physicians will be 65 or older within the next decade), the increasing prevalence of specialty care as shown in the graph on the facing page, demographics—specifically population growth and aging—and the increasing number of medically insured patients seeking health care after the Patient Protection and Affordable Care Act (ACA) went into effect in 2010. The light blue section shows the most likely range for the projected shortfall.

In recent years, the government has been providing incentives to hospitals, asking providers to take on more risk through bundled payments that extend thirty, sixty, and ninety days beyond discharge to encourage close working relationships with post-acute care facilities and home care.

According to Ukiah Valley Medical Center president Gwen Matthews, "Health care systems are being encouraged to move up the food chain, to take risks for targeted populations, which in turn provides an incentive for coordination, collaboration, and integration of care through a team of diverse professionals working together with community workers who support the promotion of health, mitigate the impact of chronic disease, and keep people from needing the high cost services."

As the saying goes, an ounce of prevention is worth a pound of cure, and those paying for health care are seeing the financial benefits of prevention and value-based care. If current trends continue, questions about how medical intervention will improve the quality of life will be asked before pills are prescribed, procedures are scheduled, and CPR is administered.

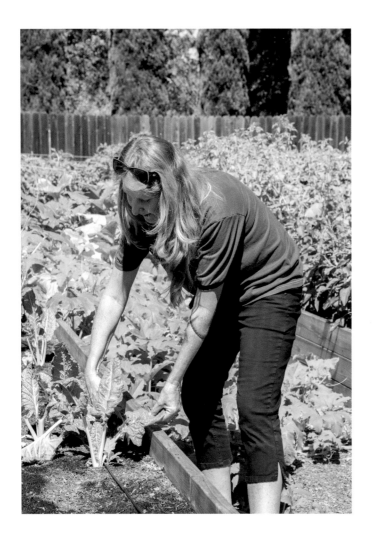

Above: North Coast Opportunities' (NCO) Tammy Alakszay tends one of the community gardens NCO supports in Mendocino and Lake Counties.

Opposite: Pictured is the mustard that springs up in front of the old barn at Testa Vineyards each year.

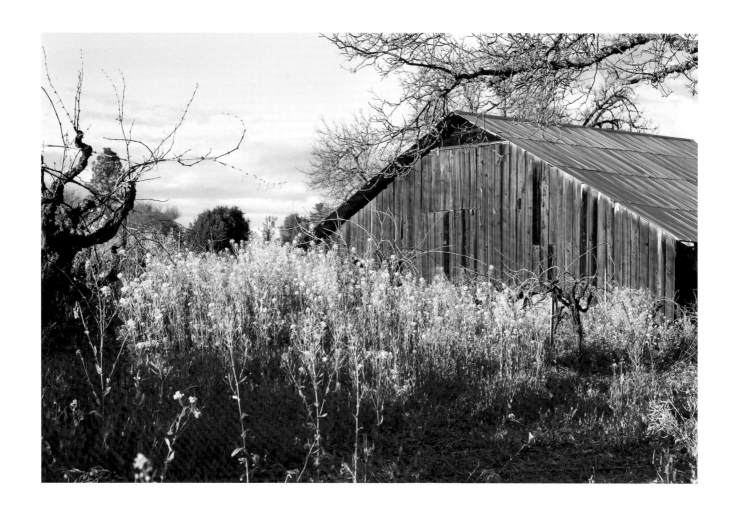

As the saying goes, an ounce of prevention is worth a pound of cure,
and those paying for health care are seeing the financial benefits of
prevention and value-based care.

APPENDIX B

Financial History of Health Care

1929 Baylor Hospital introduces a health insurance payment plan for teachers. Those who enroll pay fifty cents each month, and Baylor picks up the tab on hospital care.

1929 Blue Cross is born, based on the Baylor system of prepaid hospital care.

1930 Blue Shield develops a new medical service plan that begins providing reimbursement for physician services (as opposed to hospital care). The Blue Shield logo is developed to distinguish it from the Blue Cross hospital plan and also to show a connection to the companion hospital plan.

1943 The National War Labor Board rules that employer-based health care should be tax exempt. As employers compete for employees during World War II and immediately afterward, job-based insurance becomes a way to entice labor without running afoul of the wage freeze imposed by the government.

1954 The Revenue Act excludes an employer's contributions to health plans from taxable income. This allows employers to vie for employees using health plans, causing a huge increase in the number of people with health insurance. In 1940, only 9 percent of people had health insurance. By 1953, 63 percent had health insurance. By the 1960s, 70 percent of the population was covered by some type of private, voluntary health insurance plan.

1965 Medicare and Medicaid are enacted, extending health coverage to almost all Americans sixty-five and older, to low-income children deprived of parental support and their caretaker relatives, to the blind, and to individuals with disabilities.

1965 July 1, more than 19 million individuals enroll in Medicare.

1972 Medicare eligibility is extended to individuals under the age of sixty-five with long-term disabilities and end-stage renal disease.

1973   The HMO Act provides grants and loans to develop health maintenance organizations (HMOs). Those meeting federal guidelines for comprehensive benefits are given preferential treatment.

1981   Freedom of Choice waivers and home- and community-based care waivers are established in Medicaid; states are required to provide additional payments to hospitals treating a disproportionate share of low-income patients.

1983   An inpatient, acute hospital prospective payment system for the Medicare program based on patient diagnoses is adopted to replace cost-based payments.

1989   The resource-based, relative-value scale for physicians is established, replacing charge-based payments. Procedures are given a relative value based on geographic location and other factors.

1997   The Balanced Budget Act of 1997 includes significant reduction in provider and plan payments and creates the Sustainable Growth Rate for Physicians fees (SGR), which is designed to make sure Medicare expenses do not grow faster than the GDP. It does not work, and every year Congress makes adjustments to the SGR. This continual need to adjust the "doctor fix" leads to the SGR's repeal in in April 2015.

2003   The Medicare Prescription Drug Improvement and Modernization Act provides outpatient prescription drug benefit and establishes premiums for beneficiaries with higher incomes.

2010   The Affordable Care Act is passed, expanding Medicaid to families at 138 percent of federal poverty level. It expands prevention benefits, establishes an income-related premium for Medicare Part D, and more, slowing the growth in Medicare payments and initiating other reforms in both payment and delivery systems.

2015   Congress repeals the SGR and implements a new payment approach.

APPENDIX C

Timeline of Health Care Milestones
Text in green indicates local Ukiah milestones.

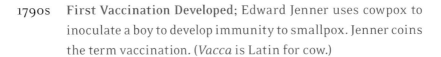

1790s   **First Vaccination Developed**; Edward Jenner uses cowpox to inoculate a boy to develop immunity to smallpox. Jenner coins the term vaccination. (*Vacca* is Latin for cow.)

1813   **US Vaccine Agency Established**; James Madison establishes the National Vaccine Agency by signing the congressionally approved "Act to Encourage Vaccination." The post office is required to carry any package of half an ounce for free if it contains smallpox vaccine material.

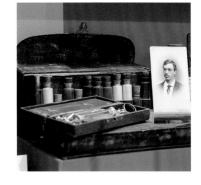

1849   **First Woman Graduates from Medical School**; Elizabeth Blackwell graduates from Geneva Medical College in Upstate New York.

1860   **First Nursing School Established**; Florence Nightingale opens the first School of Nursing at St. Thomas' Hospital in London, England.

1879   **National Board of Health Established**; The forty-fifth Congress passes "An Act to Prevent the Introduction of Infectious or Contagious Disease into the United States and to Establish a National Board of Health," creating the Board of Health.

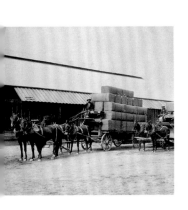

1881   Mendocino County Opens County Hospital and Farm; W. N. Moore serves as attending physician to sixty patients. The population of Ukiah is 933, according to the 1880 census.

1887   Ukiah's Cleveland Sanitarium Opens.

1889   Mendocino State Asylum for the Insane Established.

1889   **Johns Hopkins School of Nursing Established**; Johns Hopkins Hospital establishes a nursing school upon opening its hospital. As one of the earliest hospital-based nursing schools in

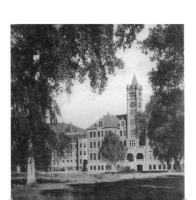

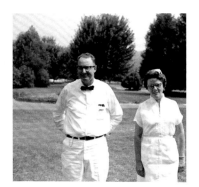

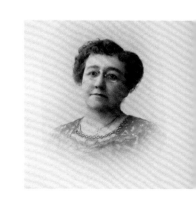

the United States, nurse leaders consult with Florence Nightingale to create the educational program. These same nurse leaders establish what will become the National League for Nursing Education and help establish the American Nurses Association.

1893   **Mendocino State Asylum for the Insane Opens;** The hospital opens December 12, 1893 with Dr. Edward Warren King as superintendent, and 150 male patients arrive from mental hospitals in Napa, Stockton, and Angus. The female wing opens in 1894. In the 1890s, this hospital is three miles from Ukiah, about a twenty-five-minute horse-and-buggy ride. Ukiah's population is 1,627, according to the 1890 census.

1895   **Wilhelm Roentgen Discovers X-rays.**

1900   **Fewer Than Five Percent of Women Give Birth in Hospitals.**

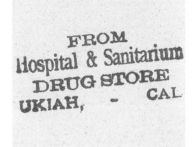

1902   **Ukiah's Dr. Ida May Lathrop Opens the Lathrop Hospital;** at a time when few female doctors are in practice, Dr. Lathrop opens her hospital on the corner of Oak and Stephenson Streets, specializing in pediatrics and women's health. Lathrop was a pioneer in her choice of profession and in her scope of practice.

1902   **Ukiah Hospital and Sanitarium Opens;** According to the *Ukiah Dispatch* dated March 14, 1902, Superintendent Dr. W. N. Moore manages the hospital, offering one-year subscriptions that "entitle the holders to…apply at the hospital for examinations, treatment, medicines and dressings all of which are furnished free on the Doctor's prescriptions. In case of illness or accidents of any kind necessitating the confinement of a member to his or her bed, they are received into the hospital where they are furnished with bed, board, medicines, dressings and a nurse together with the services of a physician at any time and as many times as necessity may demand during the entire year, all for the sum of $12.00." (This is twenty-seven years before Baylor Hospital in Dallas, Texas, opens; Baylor is widely credited as having offered the first subscription service.)

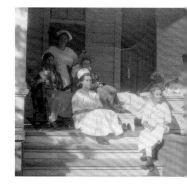

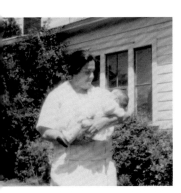

1909   **First University-Based Nursing Program Established;** The University of Minnesota offers the first Bachelor of Science in Nursing degree and graduates the first nurse with a bachelor's degree in nursing.

1914   Langland Hospital Opens; Nurse Cora Langland opens a hospital in her home on the corner of Spring and Stephenson Streets, boasting a "modern operating room."

1918   Mendocino State Asylum for the Insane renamed Mendocino State Hospital.

1921   **Insulin Used to Treat Diabetes;** Fredrick Banting and Charles Best discover insulin as a treatment for type 1 diabetes.

1923   **Yale School of Nursing Established;** Yale School of Nursing becomes the first nursing school to adopt a curriculum based on an educational plan rather than on hospital service needs; this approach is recommended by the Rockefeller Foundation-funded Goldmark Report.

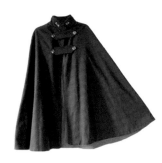

1927   Ukiah General Hospital Opens; Theresa Kramer Ray uses subscriptions (short-term loans) from community members to finance the construction of a new hospital at 564 South Dora Street.

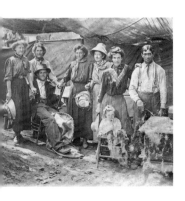

1929   **Baylor Hospital in Dallas, Texas, Sets Stage for Blue Cross Health Insurance;** Baylor implements a prepaid hospital insurance plan to help teachers afford medical care. This is the precursor to Blue Cross.

1929   **Alexander Fleming Discovers Penicillin;** While Fleming recognizes penicillin's use as a bacteria inhibitor, it is not until the 1940s that an Oxford University team led by Howard Florey produces it commercially for medical use. Ukiah's Dr. J. E. Gardner is one of the first to prescribe penicillin in Ukiah. He offers it to a man dying from pneumonia, referring to it as a new medication being used by the Army, and is thrilled when the man who, days before, was on his deathbed comes into his office as though he has hardly been ill.

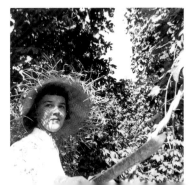

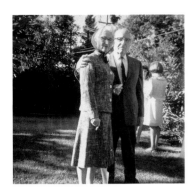

1941   Nicholas Zbitnoff Opens His Ukiah Practice.

1947   Dr. Glenn Miller Begins His Fifty-Year Career in Ukiah.

1956   Hillside Community Hospital Opens.

1956   **Columbia University School of Nursing Offers First US Master's Degree in a Clinical Nursing Specialty.**

1956   **Hill-Burton Act Established.**

1957   The new county hospital facility was completed.

1957   One of Ukiah's First Specialists Arrives in Ukiah: General Surgeon Dr. Hugh Curtis.

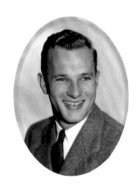

1960   **Ninety-Seven Percent of Births Occur in Hospitals;** Continuous electronic fetal monitoring is introduced.

1965   **Medicare and Medicaid Established;** President Johnson signs the Social Security Amendment of 1965, creating Medicare for the elderly and Medicaid for the poor.

1965   **The Role of Nurse Practitioner (NP) Established.**

1966   Hillside Community Hospital Becomes a Non-Profit Hospital.

1967   **Lanterman-Petris-Short Act Passed;** This act dramatically changes mental health funding in California and the United States.

1969   **Dr. Elisabeth Kübler-Ross Publishes Her Book** *On Death and Dying*; In this famous book, Kübler-Ross makes a plea for home care and advocates that families be encouraged to participate in life-altering medical decisions for the terminally ill.

1971   **Hospice Movement Begins in United States;** Florence Wald and her associates found Hospice, Inc., establishing the hospice movement in the United States.

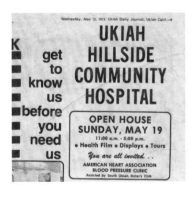

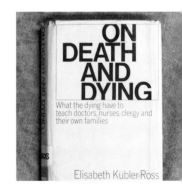

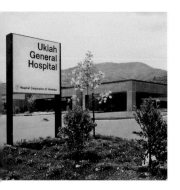

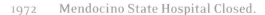

1972   Mendocino State Hospital Closed.

1975   The First Large Cohort of Specialists Arrive in Ukiah; Seven
          specialists, encouraged by Dr. Curtis, arrive in Ukiah and
          change the medical landscape of the community. They are Dr.
          Albert Baltins, orthopedic surgeon; Dr. Robert Calson, inter-
          nist and allergist; Dr. David Carter, internist and emergency
          medicine; Dr. Donald Coursey, otolaryngologist; Dr. Paul Jep-
          son, urology; Dr. Jack Mason, ophthalmology; and Dr. Vincent
          Valente, obstetrics and gynecology.

1976   New Ukiah General Hospital Opens at 1120 South Dora Street.

1978   Adventist Health Purchases Hillside Community Hospital.

1978   First Baby Born Via In-Vitro Fertilization; Louise Brown,
          conceived through in-vitro fertilization, is born on July 25 in
          Oldham, England, to Leslie and John Brown.

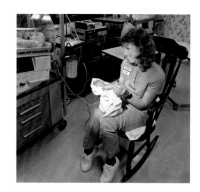

1980   Hillside Community Hospital closes its Laws Avenue facility
          and opens on Hospital Drive as Ukiah Adventist Hospital.

1982   Digital Picture Archiving System Installed in Kansas City;
          University of Kansas Medical School installs large-scale dig-
          ital imaging system so X-rays and other medical scans can be
          read digitally.

1982   Medicare Adds Hospice Care to Its Offerings.

1983   Prospective Payment System Implemented.

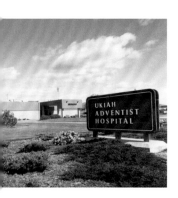

1987   AIDS Recognized as Epidemic; On July 23, President Ronald
          Reagan establishes a thirteen-member Commission on the
          Human Immunodeficiency Virus Epidemic.

1988   Ukiah Adventist Hospital Buys Assets of Ukiah General Hos-
          pital; Ukiah Adventist Hospital begins blending the assets
          and human resources, becoming the sole community hospi-
          tal. It is renamed Ukiah Valley Medical Center in 1989.

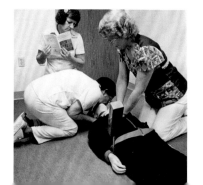

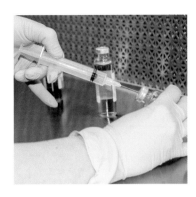

1989   **First Human Gene Transfer;** On May 22, the National Institute of Health (NIH) conducts its first gene transfer in humans. A cancer patient is infused with tumor-infiltrating lymphocytes (TIL) that have been altered by the insertion of a gene. This allows scientists to track the special cancer-fighting cells in the body to increase the understanding of TIL therapy.

1990   County Closes Mendocino Community Hospital; According to a story published in the *Ukiah Daily Journal* on August 10, 1990, "After voting two weeks ago to try to resuscitate Mendocino Community Hospital, county supervisors decided Thursday they were working on a terminally ill case and pulled the plug."

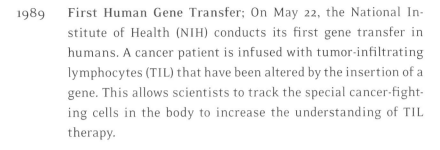

1990   **Seiji Ogawa Discovers Magnetic Resonance Imaging (MRI) Technology;** MRI technology radically changes the field of neuroscience, our understanding of the brain, and the diagnosis and treatment of mental health issues.

1992   Mendocino Community Health Clinic (MCHC) Opens; MCHC offers a seamless transition to patients who receive outpatient care from the county, setting up the clinic in the old county hospital to provide medical, behavioral, and oral health care.

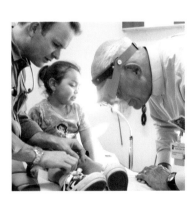

1994   **Physician-Assisted Suicide Becomes Legal;** Oregon's Death with Dignity Act passes.

1995   Ukiah Valley Primary Care (UVPC) Established; Following the trend of moving from solo to group practices, UVPC opens with four pediatricians and three family practitioners, later becoming the largest physician medical group in Ukiah.

1997   **Balanced Budget Act Reduces Reimbursement for Medical Care to Hospitals and Physicians.**

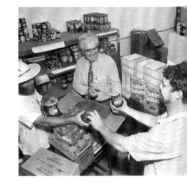

1998   Ukiah Valley Medical Center (UVMC) Birthing Center Opens.

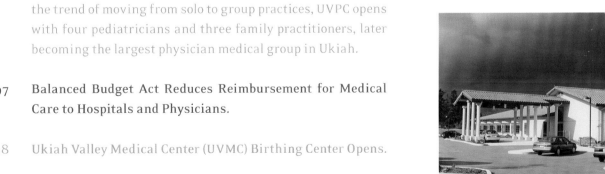

2000s   **UVMC Becomes a Smoke-Free Campus;** Believe it or not, doctors frequently smoked in the physicians' lounge throughout the 1970s and '80s. When smoking fell out of fashion, many medical providers quit, but patients continued to smoke on campus until the hospital created a smoke-free environment for everyone.

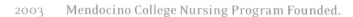

2003   Mendocino College Nursing Program Founded.

2003   **Medicare Prescription Drug, Improvement and Moderniza-tion Act Adds New Prescription Drug Benefit.**

2004   UVMC Outpatient Pavilion Lab Opens.

2005   UVMC Outpatient Pavilion Begins Surgical Services, Names Facility After Dr. Hugh P. Curtis.

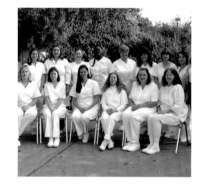

2009   **Feds Provide Financial Incentives to Adopt Electronic Medical Records**; As part of the American Recovery and Re-investment Act, Congress develops a set of incentives (e.g., $44,000 per physician) and penalties (reduced reimburse-ments to doctors who do not adopt electronic medical records by 2015) to encourage electronic medical records nationwide.

2010   **Affordable Care Act (ACA) Passes**; The ACA expands access to insurance, increases consumer protections, emphasizes prevention and wellness, improves quality and performance, thereby expanding the health workforce and curbing rising health care costs.

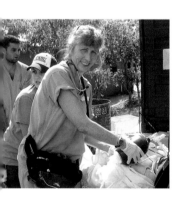

2010   **Haiti Devastated by Earthquake**; Sixty UVMC clinician volun-teers help keep a hospital open for six weeks in Port-au-Prince after the earthquake that killed thousands of Haitians.

2015   UVMC Begins Construction on New Emergency Department and Intensive Care Unit.

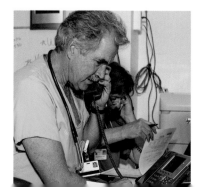

ENDNOTES

Numbers refer to endnote numbers in the text.

1. Mendocino-Lake County Medical Society, *Statement on Mendocino Community Status*, Sept. 11, 1980, 2-4.

2. H. A. Sultz and K. M. Young, *Health Care USA: Understanding Its Organization and Delivery* (Burlington, MA: Jones & Bartlett Learning, 2014), 71.

3. "Hospital Bill Passed in 1889; 65-year History," *Ukiah Daily Journal*, Nov. 19, 1954.

4. "Mendocino State Hospital Marks Mental Health Week," *Ukiah Daily Journal*, April 28, 1958.

5. Amy Brooker, assistant to the director of the Reagan Ranch, interview with Dr. Paul Jepson via email, May 6, 2015.

6. "Little Likelihood of MSH Shut-Down Seen Despite Post's Recommendations," *Ukiah Daily Journal*, Feb. 26, 1970.

7. "Open House for Public Sunday at Modern Plant," *Ukiah Daily Journal*, Oct. 12, 1956.

8. "Hospital Proposal before Board: Hillside Plans New Facility on Orchard," *Ukiah Daily Journal*, May 7, 1975.

9. "Pressure on Council Feared by Board," *Ukiah Daily Journal*, Dec. 3, 1975.

10. "Hospital Proposal," *Ukiah Daily Journal* (see endnote 8).

11. George Weisz, "The History of Medicine: Early Specialization in America" (blog), *Oxford University Press' Academic Insights for the Thinking World*, Feb. 11, 2008. Retrieved Aug. 6, 2015, from http://blog.oup.com/2008/02/specialization/.

12. Phyllis Curtis, wife of deceased general surgeon Dr. Hugh Curtis, interview with the author, March 12, 2015.

13. Marvin Trotter, internal medicine physician, quoting Dr. Gene Lapkass, interview with the author, April 14, 2015.

14. "Cadet Corps," *AAHN: American Association for the History of Nursing* website. Retrieved June 25, 2015, from https:/aahn.org/features/cadet.html.

15. Ibid.

16. Kevin Pan, "11 Ways Nursing Has Changed Since the 50s," *Mighty Nurse* website, April 13, 2014. Retrieved Aug. 20, 2015, from http://www.mightynurse.com/11-ways-nursing-has-changed-since-the-50s-stories/.

17. Karen Kelly, "Women's Leadership in the Development of Nursing," in *Gender and Women's Leadership: A Reference Handbook*, edited by Karen O'Connor (Thousand Oaks, CA: SAGE Publications, Inc., 2010), 712–720.

18. Julie Blanche, "Nursing 50 Years Back and Today," *HealtheCareers* website, Nov. 2, 2010. Retrieved June 1, 2015, from https://healthecareers.com/article/career/nursing-50-years-back-and-today-how-the-nursing-field-has-changed-over-the-last-50-years/.

19. "The Nursing Process," *ANA: American Nurses Association* website (n.d.). Retrieved June 25, 2015, from http://www.nursingworld.org/EspeciallyForYou/StudentNurses/Thenursingprocess.aspx.

20. Blanche, "Nursing" (see endnote 18).

21. Charles Tiffin, "Beyond the Bedside: The Changing Role of Today's Nurses," *Huffington Post* website, March 1, 2013. Retrieved July 23, 2015, from www.huffingtonpost.com. (TED is a non-profit organization devoted to spreading ideas; it began in 1984 as a conference where technology, entertainment, and design converged.)

22. "Hubert Humphrey," *Wikiquote*, last modified Nov. 3, 2015, https://en.wikiquote.org/wiki/Hubert_Humphrey.

23. Susan Era, retired director of Mendocino County Social Services, interview with the author, Aug. 13, 2015.

24. *Mental Health Services Act*, California Department of Health Care Services. Retrieved June 15, 2015, from http://www.dhcs.ca.gov/services/mh/Pages/MH_Prop63.aspx.

25. "1915(b) Managed Care Waivers," Medicaid.gov. Retrieved Dec. 31, 2015, from https://www.medicaid.gov.

26. Susan Baird Kanaan, "Early Lessons and Challenges from the Healthy Mendocino Community of Solution," *Journal of the American Board of Family Medicine*, vol. 26, no. 3 (2013), 316-322.

27. "Adult Obesity Facts," *Centers for Disease Control and Prevention* website. Retrieved July 10, 2015, from www.cdc.gov/obesity/data/adult.html.

28. "Field Poll: Mendocino County Voters Express Concern About Obesity," *Ukiah Daily Journal*, Jan. 25, 2013.

29. "Obesity May Shorten Life Expectancy Up To 8 Years," *McGill University Health Centre* website, Dec. 4, 2014. Retrieved Nov. 12, 2015, from https://muhc.ca/newsroom/news/obesity-may-shorten-life-expectancy-8-years/.

30. Dr. Richard Roberts, family physician and international speaker, interview with the author, June 8, 2015.

31. N. C. Doohan, J. Endres, N. Koehn, et al., "Back to the Future: Reflections on the History of the Future of Family Medicine," *Journal of the American Board of Family Medicine*, vol. 27, no. 6 (2014), 839-845.

32. Gawande, Atul, "Overkill," *The New Yorker Annals of Health Care* website, May 4, 2015. Retrieved Mar. 13, 2016, from http://www.newyorker.com/magazine/2015/05/11/overkill-atul-gawande/.

IMAGE CREDITS

All images are photographs unless otherwise specified, and are used with permission. All copyrights belong to the original photographer or contributor. We did our best to check every fact; we apologize for any errors. Numbers refer to page number in the text followed by the number of the image on that page from top to bottom, then from left to right.

o 1. Cover: Map of Ukiah, California published by W. W. Elliot, Oakland, California.

2. Front Cover: Dr. Krueger and nurse Margaret Bernard administer vaccine to a young girl. Contributed by Cindy Roper, Mendocino County Health and Human Services.

3. Back Cover: Dr. Zbitnoff. Photograph by Evan Johnson.

4. Back Cover: Jerry Chaney, circa 1971. Contributed by Jerry Chaney, RN.

5. Back Cover: A surgical team delivers a baby via cesarean section. Photograph by Evan Johnson.

6. Back Cover: Dr. John W. Hudson's case of homeopathic medicines on display at the Grace Hudson Museum. Contributed by the Grace Hudson Museum.

7. Inside Back Flap of Dust Jacket: Author Jendi Coursey, 2013. Photograph by Joe McNally.

8. Inside Back Flap of Dust Jacket: Researchers Lisa Ray and Julie Fetherston, 2016. Photograph by Jendi Coursey, Indigo Studios.

ii 1. Nelson Family Vineyards in November 2014. Photograph by Jendi Coursey, Indigo Studios.

vii 1. Sanborn Perris map of Ukiah in 1898, contributed by the Held-Poage Memorial Home and Research Library.

viii 1. Map of Ukiah, California, from *Metsker's Atlas of Mendocino County*, published by Metsker Maps. Contributed by the Held-Poage Memorial Home and Research Library.

2. Original County Hospital Buildings. Contributed by the Held-Poage Memorial Home and Research Library.

3. Dr. Ida May Lathrop-Malpus in the driver's seat. Contributed by Ed Bold.

4. Ukiah Valley Medical Center, circa 1998. Contributed by Ukiah Valley Medical Center.

5. Ukiah General Hospital, mid-1980s. Contributed by obstetrical nurse Nyota Wiles, RN.

6. Mendocino State Hospital. Original photograph by A. O. Carpenter in his book *Picturesque Mendocino*, a book authorized by the Mendocino County Board of Supervisors, published by Ukiah Republican Print. Tinted version of the image contributed by the Held-Poage Memorial Home and Research Library.

7. Hillside Community Hospital, circa 1957. Contributed by the Held-Poage Memorial Home and Research Library.

ix 1. Geographical & climatic map of the state of California compiled from actual surveys and published by the California State Board of Trade. 1888. Lith. H. S. Crocker & Co. S.F.; Image List No. 4104.001; used with permission of the David Rumsey Map Collection, www.davidrumsey.com

2. Mendocino County Courthouse, circa 1890. Contributed by the Grace Hudson Museum.

xiii 1. Ukiah Valley. Photograph by Jendi Coursey, Indigo Studios.

2 1. Dr. Ida May Lathrop-Malpus from the *History of Mendocino and Lake Counties* (1914) by A. O. Carpenter and Percy H. Millberry, contributed by the Held-Poage Memorial Home and Research Library.

2. Dr. Nicholas Zbitnoff. Contributed by the Zbitnoff family.

3. Dr. Hugh Curtis. Contributed by Dr. Curtis' widow, Phyllis Curtis.

4. Dr. Laurence Hartley. Contributed by obstetrical nurse Nyota Wiles, RN.

4 1. Jenny Jackson weaving at the Pinoleville Rancheria, 1892. Photo by Henry W. Henshaw, courtesy of the National Anthropological Archives, Smithsonian Institution. Contributed by the Grace Hudson Museum.

4   2. Pickers at a hop camp, circa 1911. Contributed by the Held-Poage Memorial Home and Research Library.

5   1. Bob Winsby picking hops on the Ford Ranch, 1914. Contributed by the Held-Poage Memorial Home and Research Library.

6   1. John Brakebill and Dr. Louise E. Petty, Mendocino State Hospital, 1965. Contributed by the Held-Poage Memorial Home and Research Library.

2. Dr. Ronald Gester in the Ukiah Valley Medical Center Emergency Room. Contributed by Ukiah Valley Medical Center.

7   1. 2014 Human Race fundraiser in Ukiah. Photograph by Jendi Coursey, Indigo Studios.

2. Lucy Soriano in front of the Ukiah Valley Medical Center Perinatal Program building. Contributed by Ukiah Valley Medical Center.

8   1. Grape harvest. Photograph by Evan Johnson.

2. Tanoak wagon. Photograph from the Sweeley-Escola Collection, contributed by the Held-Poage Memorial Home and Research Library.

3. Men shearing sheep. Photograph by A. O. Carpenter in his book *Picturesque Mendocino*, a book authorized by the Mendocino County Board of Supervisors, published by Ukiah Republican Print. Image number 2003-1-214 from the Bob Lee Collection, contributed by the Grace Hudson Museum.

9   1. Romer Vista Jersey Dairy delivery truck. Photograph from the Romer family archives, contributed by the Held-Poage Memorial Home and Research Library.

2. Hop kiln at the old McGlashan Ranch, circa 1955. Photograph from the Hayes collection, contributed by the Held-Poage Memorial Home and Research Library.

10 1. The McKinley building at the corner of State and Standley Streets, 2015. Photograph by Jendi Coursey, Indigo Studios.

2. Redemeyer vineyard, 2014. Photograph by Jendi Coursey, Indigo Studios.

11 1. Poppies along the railroad track, 2014. Photograph by Jendi Coursey, Indigo Studios.

2. Path in Low Gap Park, 2015. Photograph by Jendi Coursey, Indigo Studios.

12 1. Ruddick Family. Back row left to right: Louis, Myrtle, "Toots", Earnest. Middle row: Louis Mordecai Ruddick, unidentified boy, Rosanna Ruddick, on laps: Arch and Minnie Merle, circa 1897. Contributed by Carolyn Brown, RN. It is a photograph of her ancestors.

2. Civil War Medic Drill. Photograph 2003-1-556 from the Bob Lee Collection, contributed by the Grace Hudson Museum.

3. Drs. L. E. Van Allen & H. O. Cleland remove 52-inch cyst from Indian woman, 1914. Contributed by the Cleland family.

4. Original County Hospital Building. Contributed by the Held-Poage Memorial Home and Research Library.

5. Langland Hospital. Contributed by Ed Bold.

6. Mendocino State Hospital. Original photograph by A. O. Carpenter in his book *Picturesque Mendocino*, a book authorized by the Mendocino County Board of Supervisors, published by Ukiah Republican Print. Tinted version of the image contributed by the Held-Poage Memorial Home and Research Library.

13 1. Noni Chaney, RN. Photograph by Evan Johnson.

2. Ukiah General Hospital. Contributed by the Held-Poage Memorial Home and Research Library.

3. Thomas Nichols recovers in the ICU in 2016. Photograph by Jendi Coursey, Indigo Studios.

4. Pediatrician and internist Dr. Jorge Allende works with pediatric patient. Contributed by Mendocino Community Health Clinic.

14 1. A family makes camp during hop-picking season. Donated by M. Hetzel and contributed by the Held-Poage Memorial Home and Research Library.

2. Hop picking office. Contributed by the Cleland family.

15 1. Original County Hospital Buildings. Contributed by the Held-Poage Memorial Home and Research Library.

16 1. Groundbreaking ceremony for Mendocino County Hospital. Original *Ukiah Daily Journal* photograph by Ben Cober. Contributed by the Held-Poage Memorial Home and Research Library.

17 1. New county hospital in 1957. Contributed by the Held-Poage Memorial Home and Research Library.

2. Nurses celebrate opening day at their new county hospital facility in 1957. Contributed by the Held-Poage Memorial Home and Research Library.

18 1. A letter from the Los Angeles Knights of Pythias. Contributed by the Held-Poage Memorial Home and Research Library.

19 1. Ward 6 of the Mendocino County Hospital. Contributed by the Held-Poage Memorial Home and Research Library.

2. Map of Mendocino County Hospital. Contributed by the Held-Poage Memorial Home and Research Library.

20 1. Groundbreaking ceremony for Ukiah General Hospital. Contributed by obstetrical nurse Nyota Wiles, RN.

2. Hillside Community Hospital nursery in 1956. Contributed by Mendocino Community Health Clinic.

21 1. *Ukiah Daily Journal* front page from December 6 1979. Contributed by the Held-Poage Memorial Home and Research Library.

22 1. Three health providers. Contributed by Mendocino Community Health Clinic.

2. Dr. Bill Fisher. Contributed by Mendocino Community Health Clinic.

3. Physician Assistant Thomas Feiertag. Contributed by Mendocino Community Health Clinic.

23 1. Obstetrician and gynecologist Dr. Karen Crabtree. Photograph by Jendi Coursey, Indigo Studios.

24 1. Mendocino State Hospital, late 1800s. Photograph contributed by the Held-Poage Memorial Home and Research Library.

25 1. Superintendent of Mendocino State Hospital Dr. E. W. King, circa 1895. Contributed by the Held-Poage Memorial Home and Research Library.

26 1. Old ward of the Mendocino State Hospital. From the Ron Parker Collection, contributed by the Held-Poage Memorial Home and Research Library.

2. Beecher F. Conover and Agnes Chapman at Mendocino State Hospital, 1966. Contributed by the Held-Poage Memorial Home and Research Library.

27 1. Patients spending time outside at Mendocino State Hospital prior to 1955. Contributed by the Held-Poage Memorial Home and Research Library.

28 1. Mendocino State Hospital bus driver Robert Enright. Contributed by the Held-Poage Memorial Home and Research Library.

2. Mendocino State Hospital kitchen. Contributed by the Held-Poage Memorial Home and Research Library.

3. Tom Giles works in the Mendocino State Hospital pharmacy. Contributed by the Held-Poage Memorial Home and Research Library.

4. Andy Andrews stands next to the Mendocino State Hospital dairy sign. Contributed by the Held-Poage Memorial Home and Research Library.

29 1. Patients getting some fresh air at Mendocino State Hospital. Contributed by the Held-Poage Memorial Home and Research Library.

30 1. City of Ten Thousand Buddhas, 2015. Photograph by Jendi Coursey, Indigo Studios.

31 1. Receipt from 1921. Contributed by Ed Bold.

32 1. Ukiah 1910. Contributed by Ed Bold.

2. Hop pickers at camp, 1910. Contributed by the Held-Poage Memorial Home and Research Library.

33 1. Langland Hospital. Contributed by Ed Bold.

2. Dr. John W. Hudson's case of homeopathic medicines on display at the Grace Hudson Museum. Contributed by the Grace Hudson Museum.

34 1. Dr. Ida May Lathrop-Malpus in the driver's seat. Contributed by Ed Bold.

35 1. Theresa Ray, 1957. Contributed by Lori Watt Vest (Steve's older sister).

36 1. Ukiah General Hospital. Contributed by the Held-Poage Memorial Home and Research Library.

37 1. Ukiah General Hospital's new facility on 1120 South Dora Street. Contributed by obstetrical nurse Nyota Wiles, RN.

38 1. Nurse policy booklet. Contributed by general surgeon Dr. Larry Falk.

39 1. Ukiah General Hospital groundbreaking. Contributed by obstetrical nurse Nyota Wiles, RN.

40 1. Dr. Emery is holding the last public-assistance delivery. Photograph by Evan Johnson.

41 1. Letter regarding unionization. Contributed by obstetrical nurse Nyota Wiles, RN.

2. Pin worn by Ukiah General Hospital employees. Contributed by obstetrical nurse Nyota Wiles, RN.

42 1. Operating Room. Photograph by Tom Liden.

43 1. First Hillside Community Hospital surgery. Contributed by Mendocino Community Health Clinic.

43 2. First Hillside Community Hospital twins. Contributed by Mendocino Community Health Clinic.

44 1. Hillside Community Hospital contractors of Slater, Penner & Wilson. Contributed by Mendocino Community Health Clinic.

2. Hillside Community Hospital. Contributed by Mendocino Community Health Clinic.

45 1. Newspaper advertisement touting Hillside wages. Contributed by Jerry Chaney, RN.

46 1. *Ukiah Daily Journal* clipping of Carolyn Brown from January 27, 1969. Contributed by the Held-Poage Memorial Home and Research Library.

2. Carolyn Brown, 2016. Photograph by Jendi Coursey, Indigo Studios.

47 1. Lab Director Orlando Knittle at Hillside Community Hospital, 1971. Contributed by Jerry Chaney, RN.

2. Hillside Community Hospital nurses station, 1971. Contributed by Jerry Chaney, RN.

48 1. Eversole Mortuary, 1925. Contributed by the Held-Poage Memorial Home and Research Library.

2. Helicopter Air Ambulance. Photograph by Evan Johnson.

3. Ukiah Ambulance at Ukiah Valley Medical Center, circa 1988. Contributed by Ukiah Valley Medical Center.

49 1. Ukiah Valley Medical Center president Gwen Matthews on a CALSTAR helicopter, 2013. Photograph by Jendi Coursey, Indigo Studios.

2. Chuck Yates with pediatric patient. Photograph by Evan Johnson.

50 1. Kaz Kazmierzak at Ukiah Valley Medical Center. Photograph by Evan Johnson.

2. Rosa Rojas, Ukiah Valley Medical Center housekeeper. Photograph by Evan Johnson.

3. Frank Walker in Ukiah Valley Medical Center Lab. Photograph by Evan Johnson.

51 1. Ukiah Valley Medical Center Emergency Room nurse Edrina Kolling. Photograph by Evan Johnson.

2. A surgical team delivers a baby via cesarean section. Photograph by Evan Johnson.

52 1. Dr. Dale Morrison. Photograph by Jendi Coursey, Indigo Studios. Contributed by Ukiah Valley Medical Center.

53 1. ValGene Devitt. Photograph by Evan Johnson.

2. Radiologist at Ukiah Valley Medical Center. Photograph by Tom Liden.

54 1. Transcriptionist at Ukiah Valley Medical Center. Photograph by Evan Johnson.

55 1. Terry Burns at Ukiah Valley Medical Center volunteer luncheon. Contributed by Ukiah Valley Medical Center.

56 1. Medical office building under construction. Contributed by Ukiah Valley Medical Center.

2. Surgery suite at Ukiah Valley Medical Center. Contributed by Ukiah Valley Medical Center.

57 1. Gwen Matthews. Photograph by Jendi Coursey, Indigo Studios.

58 1. Rural Health Center. Contributed by Ukiah Valley Medical Center.

59 1. Rendering of planned hospital renovation. Contributed by Ukiah Valley Medical Center.

2. Outpatient Pavilion Lobby. Contributed by Ukiah Valley Medical Center.

60 1. Chaplain Mary Casler in patient room. Contributed by Ukiah Valley Medical Center.

2. Mary's Rock. Photograph by Jendi Coursey, Indigo Studios.

61 1. Kathy Smith, LVN, Materiels Management Director. Contributed by Ukiah Valley Medical Center.

2. Bridget Sholin. Contributed by Ukiah Valley Medical Center.

62 1. Dr. Iyad Hanna and Richard Selzer. Contributed by Ukiah Valley Medical Center.

2. Nurses at trauma training event. Contributed by Ukiah Valley Medical Center.

3. Terry Burns and Tom Allman. Contributed by Ukiah Valley Medical Center.

63 1. Dr. Tony Burris in Wound Care. Contributed by Ukiah Valley Medical Center.

2. Wound Care technicians Rocio Barajas and Lacey Rodgers. Contributed by Ukiah Valley Medical Center.

64 1. General Practitioner Dr. Jonathan Earl Gardner. Contributed by grandson Earl Aagaard.

2. Orthopedic surgeon Dr. Kenneth Hoek with patient Jordan Smith, 2004. Photograph by Suzette Cook. Contributed by the Hoek family.

3. Ophthalmologist Dr. Randall Woesner. Contributed by Ukiah Valley Medical Center.

4. Family Medicine Practitioner Dr. Miriam "Ida" Harris. Contributed by Ukiah Valley Medical Center.

66. 1. Pigs raised at the Mendocino State Hospital. Contributed by the Held-Poage Memorial Home and Research Library.

2. Walter Freeman cares for the pigs at Mendocino State Hospital. Contributed by the Held-Poage Memorial Home and Research Library.

67 1. From the *History of Mendocino and Lake Counties California*, (1914) by A. O. Carpenter and Percy H. Millberry, contributed by the Held-Poage Memorial Home and Research Library.

68 1. Dr. Vest's children. Photograph by Jendi Coursey, Indigo Studios.

2. Reprinted from *9 Voices: The Childhood of a Family*, with permission from the Wilson family.

69 1. Logging truck, circa 1923. Contributed by the Held-Poage Memorial Home and Research Library.

2. Goudge Kiln. Contributed by the Held-Poage Memorial Home and Research Library.

3. Savings Bank of Mendocino County, circa 1956. Contributed by the Held-Poage Memorial Home and Research Library.

70 1. Dr. Eugene Lapkass. Contributed by his widow, Maiga Lapkass.

71 1. Dr. Zbitnoff. Photograph by Evan Johnson.

72 1. Rea family. Contributed by Sally Rea and Blair Johnson Carlson.

73 1. Dr. James Massengill, his wife Josie and their five children. Contributed by Karena Massengill.

74 1. Dr. Glenn Miller. Contributed by Ukiah Valley Medical Center.

75 1. Dr. Donald Coursey and his wife Lynda. Contributed by the Coursey family.

2. Drs. Jepson and Blackwelder and their wives. Contributed by the Coursey family.

76 1. Dr. Hugh Curtis with a recently caught fish. Contributed by Dr. Larry Falk.

77 1. Dr. Hugh Curtis writing surgery report. Photograph by Evan Johnson.

78 1. Hugh Curtis Surgery Center. Photograph by Jendi Coursey, Indigo Studios.

79 1. Specialists who arrived in 1976. Photograph by Jendi Coursey, Indigo Studios.

2. Marty Lombardi. Photograph by Jendi Coursey, Indigo Studios.

80 1. Orthopedic surgeon Dr. Albert Baltins. Contributed by Ukiah Valley Medical Center.

81 1. Orthopedic surgeons Dr. Albert Baltins and Dr. Tom Kilkenny. Contributed by Ukiah Valley Medical Center.

2. Pathologist Dr. Herschel Gordon and general surgeon Dr. Larry Falk. Photograph by Jendi Coursey, Indigo Studios.

82 1. Pediatrician Dr. Richard Miller. Contributed by obstetrical nurse Nyota Wiles, RN.

2. Pediatrician Dr. Sidney Maurer. Contributed by obstetrical nurse Nyota Wiles, RN.

2. Nurses and volunteers. Contributed by Ukiah Valley Medical Center.

111 1. Daniel Jenkins. Contributed by Daniel Jenkins.

112 1. First Mendocino College nurse graduates, 2004. Contributed by Mendocino College.

2. Jene Lowater, nurse graduate. Contributed by Mendocino College.

113 1. Jerry Chaney speaks at dedication ceremony for Mendocino Community Health Clinic's Fisher Building. Photograph by Jendi Coursey, Indigo Studios.

114 1. Jerry Chaney, circa 1971. Contributed by Jerry Chaney, RN.

115 1. Heather Van Housen. Photograph by Jendi Coursey, Indigo Studios.

116 1. Dr. and Mrs. H. O. Cleland. Contributed by the Cleland family.

2. Ophthalmologist Dr. Geoffrey Rice treats patient during 1995 mission trip to Nepal. Contributed by Ukiah Valley Medical Center.

3. Dr. Marvin Trotter and Carol Mordhorst. Contributed by Dr. Marvin Trotter.

4. Health care providers and members of law enforcement. Contributed by Ukiah Valley Medical Center.

118 1. Dr. H. O. Cleland in 1914. Contributed by the Cleland family.

119 1. Dr. H. O. Cleland with his family. Contributed by the Cleland family.

120 1. Dr. Krueger and nurse Margaret Bernard administer vaccine to a young girl. Contributed by Cindy Roper, Mendocino County Health and Human Services.

121 1. Dennis Denny. Contributed by the Denny family.

122 1. *Ukiah Daily Journal* front page article on December 4, 1979. Contributed by the Held-Poage Memorial Home and Research Library.

123 1. Denny family in the 1980s. Contributed by the Denny family.

124 1. Redwood Empire Fair Memory Lane Memorial. Photograph by Jendi Coursey, Indigo Studios.

125 1. Myrna Ogelsby. Photograph by Jendi Coursey, Indigo Studios.

126 1. MCAVHN, 2016. Photograph by Jendi Coursey, Indigo Studios.

2. MCAVHN's Libby Guthrie and Cynthia Rattey, 2016. Photograph by Jendi Coursey, Indigo Studios.

127 1. Carol Mordhorst, 2016. Photography by Jendi Coursey, Indigo Studios.

128 1. Mendocino County Community Health Status Report 2004. Contributed by Mendocino County Health and Human Services.

129 1. Pacific Ambulance. Contributed by Ukiah Valley Medical Center.

130 1. Trauma Drill, 2015. Photograph by Peter Armstrong.

131 1. Peggy Smart at Bike Fashion Show, 2011. Photograph by Jendi Coursey, Indigo Studios.

132 1. Holly Smith at Manzanita Services, 2016. Photograph by Jendi Coursey, Indigo Studios.

2. Tapestry Family Services, 2016. Photograph by Jendi Coursey, Indigo Studios.

133 1. Tesla Talbot at Redwood Community Services, 2016. Photograph by Jendi Coursey, Indigo Studios.

134 1. The Bonita House. Photograph by Jendi Coursey, Indigo Studios.

135 1. Psychiatrist Dr. Douglas Rosoff. Contributed by the Held-Poage Memorial Home and Research Library.

136 1. *Ukiah Daily Journal* clipping from January 17, 2002. Contributed by the Held-Poage Memorial Home and Research Library.

137 1. County building at 860 North Bush Street. Photograph by Jendi Coursey, Indigo Studios.

138 1. Partnership HealthPlan of California logo. Contributed by Partnership HealthPlan of California.

139 1. Claire Teske, RN, Medical Manager, Sheriff Tom Allman, Teresa Brassfield, RN, Behavioral Court Case Manager, Robert Hurley, RN, Mental Health Nurse, and Captain Tim Pearce, Jail Commander. Teske, Brassfield and Hurley work for California Forensic Medical Group, the group contracted

to provide health care in the jails. Contributed by Ukiah Valley Medical Center.

139 2. Sheriff Tom Allman and community member Ed Keller. Photograph by Jendi Coursey, Indigo Studios.

140 1. Stacey Cryer, 2016. Photograph by Jendi Coursey, Indigo Studios.

141 1. County gaps analysis meeting, 2011. Photograph by Jendi Coursey, Indigo Studios.

142 1. Sandy O'Ferrall, 2016. Photograph by Jendi Coursey, Indigo Studios.

143 1. Ukiah Recovery Center, 2015. Photograph by Jendi Coursey, Indigo Studios.

2. Ford Street Project Executive Director Jacque Williams talks with *Ukiah Daily Journal* reporter Adam Randall at Ukiah Recovery Center, 2015. Photograph by Jendi Coursey, Indigo Studios.

144 1. Lab technician Kimi Oliveira, circa 1999. Contributed by Ukiah Valley Medical Center.

2. Medical Imaging Director Steve Daugherty, circa 1999. Contributed by Ukiah Valley Medical Center.

3. Cardiologist Dr. David Ploss. Contributed by Ukiah Valley Medical Center.

4. Emergency Room physician Dr. Charlie Evans, 2016. Photograph by Jendi Coursey, Indigo Studios.

146 1. Diabetes Educators Brenda Hoek, RN, and Linda Ayotte, RD. Photograph by Jendi Coursey, Indigo Studios.

147 1. Medical equipment, 2016. Photograph by Evan Johnson.

2. Nurse Avelina Pottinger reviews hemodialysis data, 2016. Photograph by Evan Johnson.

148 1. Radiologist Dr. Laura Winkle dictates her report while reviewing digital images, 2016. Photograph by Jendi Coursey, Indigo Studios.

2. Physician Assistant Lisa Gamble dictates patient data into the electronic medical record, 2016. Photograph by Jendi Coursey, Indigo Studios.

149 1. Critical care specialist Dr. James Gude. Contributed by Dr. James Gude.

150 1. Nurses Iva Jo Otto, RN, and Ron Pike, RN, 2016. Photograph by Jendi Coursey, Indigo Studios.

2. Family Medicine Practitioner Dr. Andrew Coren, 2016. Photograph by Jendi Coursey, Indigo Studios.

151 1. Family Medicine Practitioner Dr. Lynne Coen, 2016. Photograph by Jendi Coursey, Indigo Studios.

152 1. Dr. Richard Roberts, Dr. Mimi Doohan, and Dr. Charlie Evans, 2015. Photograph by Jendi Coursey, Indigo Studios.

153 1. Rural Health Rocks poster. Contributed by Dr. Mimi Doohan.

154 1. Gene Parsons, 2016. Photograph by Steve Eberhard.

155 1. Ukiah Valley Medical Center mission. Photograph by Jendi Coursey, Indigo Studios.

156 1. Ukiah Valley Medical Center chapel. Photograph by Jendi Coursey, Indigo Studios.

2. William Kidd and Mike Dobbs Photograph by Jendi Coursey, Indigo Studios.

157 1. Nancy Bray, RN, with Natalie Shepard. Photograph by Jendi Coursey, Indigo Studios.

2. Kittie Hawk, 2016. Photograph by Jendi Coursey, Indigo Studios.

158 1. Widow Elise Wilkins, RN, hugs her daughter while they pay their respects to husband and father Dane Wilkins, 2016. Photograph by Jendi Coursey, Indigo Studios.

159 1. Empty hospital bed, 2016. Photograph by Jendi Coursey, Indigo Studios.

160 1. Family Medicine Practitioner Dr. Robert Werra, 2016. Photograph by Jendi Coursey, Indigo Studios.

2. Hospice of Ukiah, 2016. Photograph by Jendi Coursey, Indigo Studios.

161 1. In-home care. Photograph by Evan Johnson.

162 1. *Ukiah Daily Journal* clipping from March 20, 1980, contributed by the Held-Poage Memorial Home and Research Library.

163 1. California Senator Barry Keene in *Ukiah Daily Journal* clipping from May 16, 1974. Contributed by the Held-Poage Memorial Home and Research Library.

164 1. In-home care. Photograph by Evan Johnson.

2. In-home care. Photograph by Evan Johnson.

165 1. Ukiah Valley Medical Center's Palliative Care Team: Lynn Meadows, PA; Debbie Summit, RN; Mark Apfel MD; Faith Dayton, MSW; Dominique Chevalier-Welch, Lynn Chevalier, Susan Pollesel, ST, Patti Ridella, RN. Contributed by Ukiah Valley Medical Center.

2. Speech Pathologist Susan Pollesel, 2016. Photograph by Jendi Coursey, Indigo Studios.

166 1. Ukiah Valley Medical Center Emergency Room, 2016. Photograph by Jendi Coursey, Indigo Studios.

167 1. Physician Orders for Life-Sustaining Treatment (POLST) form. Contributed by the Coalition for Compassionate Care of California, a statewide partnership of regional and statewide organizations and individuals dedicated to the advancement of palliative medicine and end-of-life care in California.

168 1. A mother pulls back her son's hair while waiting for Plowshares to open in 2015. Photograph by Jendi Coursey, Indigo Studios.

169 1. Leanna Sweet, RN, at Plowshares Peace and Justice Center of Ukiah, 2015. Photograph by Jendi Coursey, Indigo Studios.

2. Wellness Coach Michelle Flowers explains benefits available to a woman at Plowshares Peace and Justice Center of Ukiah, 2015. Photograph by Jendi Coursey, Indigo Studios.

3. Wellness Coach Michelle Flowers poses with a man at Plowshares Peace and Justice Center of Ukiah, 2015. Photograph by Jendi Coursey, Indigo Studios.

4. Leanna Sweet, RN, checks blood pressure at Plowshares Peace and Justice Center of Ukiah, 2015. Photograph by Jendi Coursey, Indigo Studios.

170 1. Dr. Jim Withers and Dr. Mimi Doohan on School Street in Ukiah, 2015. Photograph by Jendi Coursey, Indigo Studios.

171 1. Cassell brothers. Contributed by Scott Cassell.

172 1. Scott Cassell. Contributed by the Cassell family.

2. Scott Cassell. Contributed by the Cassell family.

173 1. Mendocino Coast. Photograph by Jendi Coursey, Indigo Studios.

174 1. Theresa Lund, RN, updates a patient chart. Photograph by Evan Johnson.

176 1. Rainbow over Lake Mendocino, 2010. Photograph by Jendi Coursey, Indigo Studios.

178 1. Chart design by Colored Horse Studios. Data from "IHS Inc., The Complexities of Physician Supply and Demand: Projections from 2013 to 2025."

179 1. Chart design by Colored Horse Studios. Data from the California Health Care Foundation Almanac titled, "California Physicians: Surplus or Scarcity," published in March 2014.

180 1. Tammy Alakszay tends NCO Community Garden, 2013. Photograph by Jendi Coursey, Indigo Studios.

181 1. Testa Vineyards Barn, 2014. Photograph by Jendi Coursey, Indigo Studios.

184 1. Grape harvest at Cummiskey Station, circa 1906. Photograph from Martha Gustafson. Contributed by the Held-Poage Memorial Home and Research Library.

2. Howard Brooks transporting a wagon load of hops in front of the warehouse at the railroad in Ukiah, 1913. Contributed by the Held-Poage Memorial Home and Research Library.

3. Medical supplies used by Dr. John Hudson. Contributed by the Grace Hudson Museum.

4. Mendocino State Hospital. Contributed by the Held-Poage Memorial Home and Research Library.

185 1. Beecher F. Conover and Agnes Chapman at Mendocino State Hospital, 1966. Contributed by the Held-Poage Memorial Home and Research Library.

2. A stamp from a turn-of-the-century hospital & sanitarium in Ukiah. Contributed by the Held-Poage Memorial Home and Research Library.

3. Dr. Ida May Lathrop-Malpus from the History of Mendocino and Lake Counties by Carpenter (1914) contributed by the Held-Poage Memorial Home and Research Library.

4. Langland Hospital. Contributed by Ed Bold.

186 1. Nurse holds baby at Langland Hospital. Contributed by Ed Bold.

186 2. A family makes camp during hop-picking season. Contributed by the Held-Poage Memorial Home and Research Library.

3. Nurse's cape. Public domain photograph.

186 4. Patricia Hetzel Smith picks hops. Contributed by the Held-Poage Memorial Home and Research Library.

187 1. Dr. and Mrs. H. O. Cleland. Contributed by the Cleland family.

2. Advertisement about Hillside Community Hospital open house from the *Ukiah Daily Journal*, May 15, 1974. Contributed by Ukiah Valley Medical Center.

3. General surgeon Dr. Hugh Curtis. Contributed by widow Phyllis Curtis.

4. Dr. Elisabeth Kübler-Ross' *On Death and Dying.* Photograph by Jendi Coursey, Indigo Studios.

188 1. General Hospital. Contributed by obstetrical nurse Nyota Wiles, RN.

2. Ukiah Adventist Hospital. Contributed by Ukiah Valley Medical Center.

3. Obstetrical nurse rocks baby in Ukiah Valley Medical Center nursery. Photograph by Evan Johnson.

4. CPR Training. Contributed by Ukiah Valley Medical Center.

189 1. Gloved hands hold syringe. Contributed by Ukiah Valley Medical Center.

2. Dr. Jorge Allende and Dr. Richard McClintock examine pediatric patient. Contributed by Mendocino Community Health Clinic.

3. ValGene Devitt at a local food bank. Photograph by Evan Johnson.

4. Newly constructed Family Birth Center. Contributed by Ukiah Valley Medical Center.

190 1. Ukiah Valley Medical Center Outpatient Pavilion. Contributed by Ukiah Valley Medical Center.

2. Beth Cabral in Haiti after the 2010 earthquake. Contributed by Ukiah Valley Medical Center.

3. First Mendocino College nurse graduates, 2004. Contributed by Mendocino College.

4. Dr. Charlie Evans and Dr. Gerry Lazzareschi dictating in the Ukiah Valley Medical Center Emergency Room, 2016. Photograph by Jendi Coursey, Indigo Studios.

209 1. Author Jendi Coursey, 2013. Photograph by Joe McNally.

2. Researchers Lisa Ray and Julie Fetherston, 2016. Photograph by Jendi Coursey, Indigo Studios.

210 1. Ukiah High School Staff, 1909. Contributed by Carolyn Brown, RN.

2. Ukiah High School Yearbook Cover, 1909. Contributed by Carolyn Brown, RN.

INDEX

Page numbers in *italics* refer to images.

PUBLICATION CREDITS

Research, Lisa Ray and Julie Fetherston

Contemporary photography, Evan Johnson and Jendi Coursey; for other photography credits, see image credits section of the appendix

Initial copyediting, Jessica Vineyard, Red Letter Editing

Design, typesetting, and additional copyediting, Theresa Whitehill, Adrienne Simpson, and Lillian Rubie, Colored Horse Studios, Ukiah, California

Indexing, Peter Brigaitis and Marie Nuchols, Indexing Pros

Proofreading, Lisa Ray and Colored Horse Studios

Printing and bindery, Friesens, Canada, through Spectrum Print Group

Perseverance and Passion was typeset in Eidetic Neo, with titling in Curwen Poster and captions in MTT Milano and was printed on 100# Garda Silk White text. The book was smythe-sewn, with the hard cover edition bound in cloth over boards and wrapped in a dust jacket.

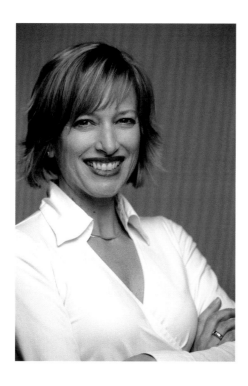

ABOUT THE AUTHOR

Jendi Coursey is a writer and photographer based in Ukiah, California. She has worked in health care communications much of her career, serving as a marketing director for Ukiah Valley Medical Center and Mendocino Community Health Clinic, as well as a public relations consultant for Mendocino County Health and Human Services and Frank R. Howard Memorial Hospital.

As the mother of a cancer survivor, the daughter of a clinical psychologist, the daughter-in-law of an otolaryngologist, and a long-time board member for the Cancer Resource Centers of Mendocino County, she appreciates health care from many perspectives, and she uses that appreciation to wonderful effect in this brief history of health care in Ukiah.

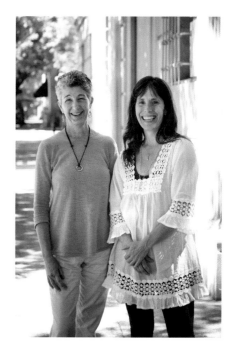

Special thanks to researchers Lisa Ray and Julie Fetherston for their humor and grace, and for their unwavering dedication to unearthing the history of health care in their hometown.

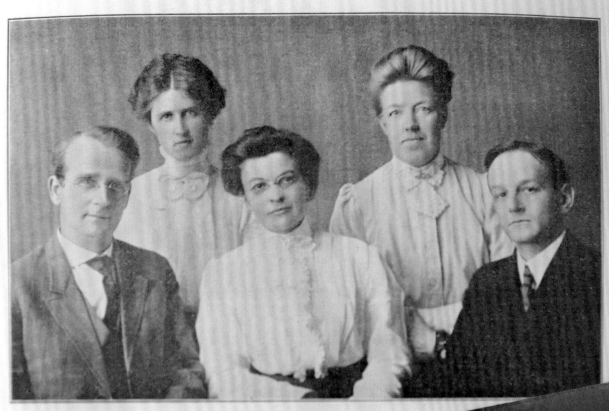

FACULTY

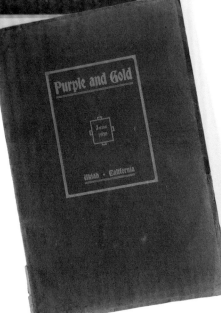